CRAFTS FOR THE DISABLED

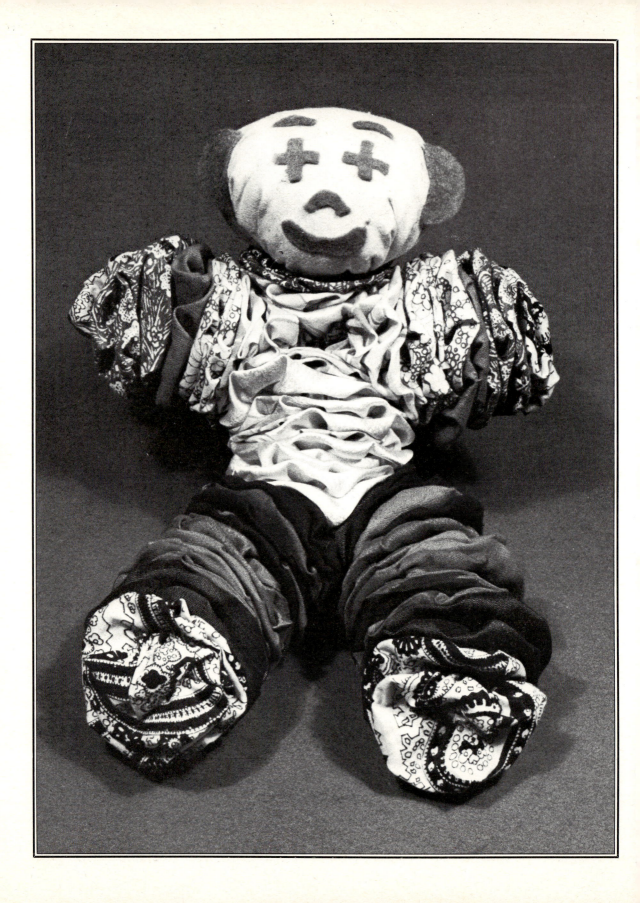

CRAFTS FOR THE DISABLED

by
Elizabeth Gault and Susan Sykes

THOMAS Y. CROWELL, PUBLISHERS
ESTABLISHED 1834
NEW YORK

ACKNOWLEDGEMENTS

We would like to express our appreciation and offer many thanks to the following: the members of the Alfred Morris Day Centre, the Ladywell Day Centre, the Woodpecker Day Centre and the Marden Court Residential Home for the inspiration to write this book; the staff for their support during our many hours spent teaching there; the Frobisher, Catford, Woolwich and Greenwich Adult Education Institutes under whose auspices the various craft classes for the handicapped where we have gained our teaching experience are run; Mary Sykes for reviving her typing skills for us; Lewis Gabriel and Gavin Gault, who have given unfailing support and encouragement; and to Bernard Schofield for his help and advice.

We would like to thank the following for allowing us to use photographs of their work in the book: Rosina Blackman (canvas embroidery rug, *33*, Chapter 1), Mrs Harris (striped jumper, *9*, Chapter 3), Joan Burton (shawl, *21*, Chapter 3), Doris Oakley (crochet bag on wooden handles, *33*, Chapter 5) and Emma Francis and Anne Meakin (knitted bag on wooden handles, *36*, Chapter 5).

Drawings by Steven Crisp; photographs by Ronald Kass, except for the following: Chapter 1, *38* and Chapter 3, *2–6b* and *11–17b* by Bill Toomey; Chapter 4, *3–12, 16* and *17* by Lewis Gabriel.

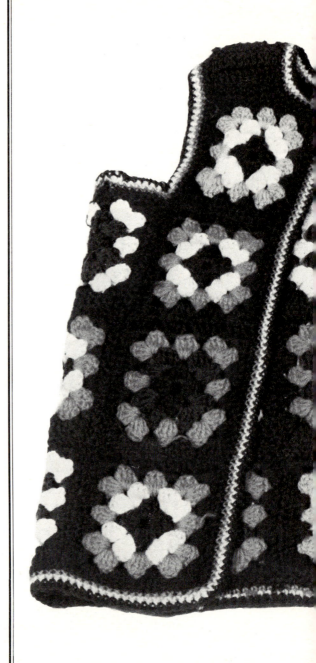

Library of Congress Cataloging in Publication Data

Gault, Elizabeth.
Crafts for the disabled.
1. Handicraft for the physically handicapped.
I. Sykes, Susan, joint author. II. Title.
TT149.G38   1979   745.5′02′40816   78-20625

ISBN 0-690-01806-1
ISBN 0-690-01825-8 pbk

CONTENTS

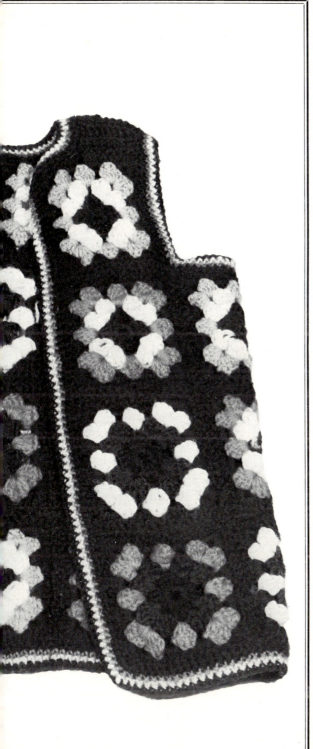

Introduction vi

1 CANVAS EMBROIDERY 1
Materials 2 – How to embroider fourteen different stitches 3 – Ideas on what to make 7 – Choosing a design 7 – Putting your design into practice 10 – Hints on working 14 – Making up and finishing 16 – Instructions for embroidering a six-colour rug 19 – a table mat 22 – a small shoulder bag 24

2 SOFT TOYS 27
Tools and equipment 28 – Materials 30 – Basic techniques 30 – Instructions for making animals from material scraps 32 – (a cat, dog, rabbit or pig) 33 – How to make glove puppets (a penguin, elephant, frog or mouse) 37 – How to make a teddy or panda 47 – How to make and dress rag dolls 55

3 KNITTING AND CROCHET 65
Equipment and materials 66 – Simple knitting techniques 66 – How to make a knitted shopping bag 69 – a child's multi-coloured jumper 70 – a child's two-colour striped jumper 70 – Instructions for working six crochet stitches 72 – Making and joining up crochet squares 74 – How to make a crochet purse 76 – a shawl 78 – a hat 79 – a child's top 80

4 CHAIR CANING 83
Materials 84 – Preparing an old chair for recaning 86 – How to cane a square stool 86 – Using beading to finish off 93 – Working other shapes 94 – Hints on working 95 – Other patterns for caning 96

5 COILS, CIRCLES AND SQUARES 99
Equipment and materials 100 – How to make French knitting tubes and plaited lengths 101 – Instructions for making a plaited oval rag rug 102 – a French knitting round rug 103 – a coiled purse 103 – a shoulder bag 104 – table mats 105 – Making material rosettes and crochet circles 105 – How to make a baby's ball 106 – a caterpillar 106 – a clown 107 – Using squares of knitting and crochet to make soft play bricks 108 – a purse 109 – a knitted or crochet bag with wooden handles 110 – a child's waistcoat 112 – a cushion cover 114

Further useful information United Kingdom 115 – United States 117

INTRODUCTION

This book has grown out of a need that we as teachers and many of our students have felt for a practical book about crafts with specific reference to the problems of disabled people. Disability, from whatever source, often brings with it a sense of loss of worth, both to the disabled person and in colouring the attitudes of those around. The common idea of what craft activity has to offer disabled people often reinforces this, with the attitude that whatever is produced, while very 'nice', is the superfluous product of a somewhat superfluous activity. As two people who have taught crafts to men and women with varying degrees of disability in day centres, adult education classes and old people's homes for some years, we both know how untrue this is. The high standard of design and manufacture of articles that many of the people we have taught have achieved, a very few of which we have been able to show in this book, confirms this, particularly with people who have never tried making anything for themselves before. Craft work can be a means of bringing out undeveloped creative potential in people whether they are disabled or not.

There are many books written in depth about various crafts as well as books about coping with disability. Here we give basic craft techniques adapted for people suffering from varying degrees of disability. We have included the simple crafts of knitting, crochet, making soft toys, chair caning and canvas embroidery, using the successful methods that have evolved from our work with disabled people. We have given clear instructions, assuming that the person who is attempting the task has never tried to do anything like it before. As well as being aimed at disabled people themselves who are interested in doing any of the crafts that we have written about, this book should be of interest to other teachers, relatives and friends of disabled people or staff in residential homes or day centres.

We haven't been concerned with the specific causes of disabilities as people can become disabled for a variety of reasons. A stroke, car accident or congenital handicap could all be causes of partial paralysis, for example. What does vary is the degree of handicap that a person experiences as a result of their disability. A person who has been very physically active would probably find a loss of mobility more of a handicap than someone who has led a sedentary way of life.

What we look at in this book are the effects of various disabilities such as lack of mobility, lack of sight, lack of sensation, lack of grip or lack of coordination. All these things can affect a person with varying degrees of severity and in various combinations, temporarily or permanently. For example many elderly people experience minor disabilities such as failing eyesight or arthritic joints and their abilities can perhaps vary from one day to the next. With some diseases a person's disabilities can increase as time passes and enthusiasm for doing a craft can obviously be affected by constant pain or the side effects of drugs which have been prescribed to control their condition. Because of this, concentration, mood and memory can all be liable to sudden or extreme changes and in teaching disabled people we feel it is important to take account of this with each individual student.

If a person has done craft work before it will have a bearing on their expertise and one craft can often be substituted for another where the onset of disability means they are no longer able to pursue their original activity. For example, someone who has been an expert knitter may find it frustrating to do knitting with a modified technique but might get a lot of satisfaction from learning a completely new craft and gaining a similar level of expertise. Whether this book is used by individuals or as a teaching aid it is important to understand the basic principles of a craft before moving on to more complicated patterns.

As most crafts entail sitting for a considerable time in one position a good working environment is essential. Lighting should be natural if possible and a seat by a window enables a person doing close work to look up and rest the eyes occasionally. If this isn't feasible and only artificial lighting is available it is best to sit directly under the light or have an angle-poise lamp directed onto the work. Good ventilation and a comfortable seat are important too and leg rests are often a help. The working surface should be at a comfortable height and should be a substantial table that won't wobble or rock. If working from a wheelchair, a bench fixed to a wall avoids problems with table legs. There are small cantilevered tables available which can be used from an armchair or wheelchair which are portable and also adjustable for height. Apart from the working surface it may be necessary to have another space nearby to put materials on. It is helpful to keep materials within easy reach and to keep the working area uncluttered. Where possible work should be left out so it can be continued at any time.

Everyone has their own way of working and a disabled person often needs to work in a very individual way, with or without manufactured aids. What is a successful method of working for a particular person can often appear to be very awkward. In the end it will be an individual's decision what he or she attempts but we feel that it shouldn't be too demanding physically so that energy can be concentrated on the good craftsmanship and design of the work. It is a good idea to try out a small example of a new or different craft to find out whether the techniques are suitable for the individual concerned and, as in attempting anything new, a degree of patience is required at the beginning! We have found from personal experience that to set oneself a mammoth task can mean becoming frustrated and bored at the lack of progress. Tiredness will also lead to mistakes so rather than working for too long at a time it is better to take a break and return later with revived enthusiasm. When errors are made it is best to rectify them otherwise they will eventually detract from the satisfaction of a well made piece of work. Ignoring a fault will often cause complications later on and lead to the work being abandoned unfinished. Undoing the work back to the point where the mistake was made can even help in the complete understanding of a technique.

When people are restricted in their movements, there can be long spells of inactivity and this applies particularly in residential situations where staff/resident ratios are high. Doing crafts as an individual activity can play an important part in alleviating the boredom that many people experience as a result, and in a home or hospital several people can work together on one article. People's abilities often complement one another and someone who is severely afflicted will be encouraged by contributing something towards a more complex finished article.

We have divided the book into chapters covering five crafts, with detailed instructions and illustrations for making finished articles which are given in order of complexity for each craft. At the beginning of each chapter there is a list of materials and equipment. We have tried to keep the special gadgetry to a minimum, using easily available household items where possible, but some people may need help in obtaining the necessary equipment and materials. There is a list of stockists at the back of the book, and many of them offer a mail-order service.

Our ultimate aim is to help disabled people become independent in the practice of the crafts described in the following pages. Well-meaning people will often take over a piece of work from a disabled person who appears slow or awkward and though this brings the short-term benefit of a quickly-finished piece of work, the long-term gain of being able to practise a craft well and independently is lost. It is for people who want to do this that this book is written. Above all we hope that it is a starting point, both for people who practise the crafts who can go on to work from more specialised books relating to crafts, and for other people who we hope will be encouraged to produce more ideas about crafts adapted to the needs of the disabled.

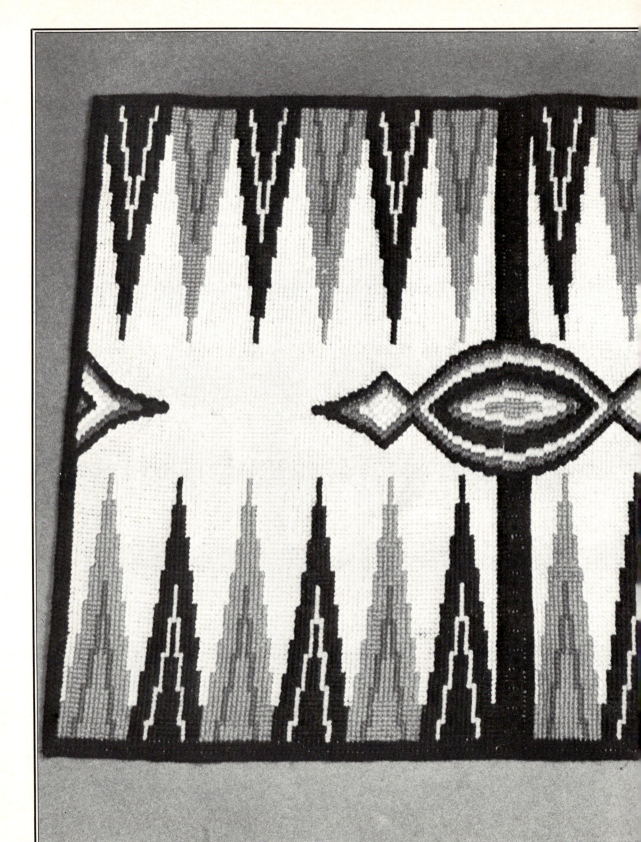

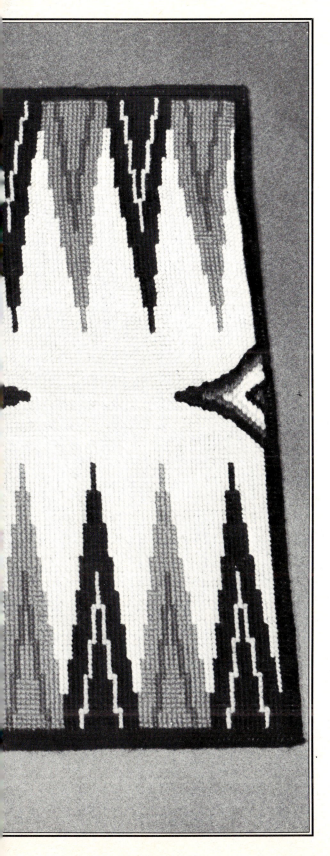

1 Canvas Embroidery

Canvas embroidery is known by several names. One of these is needlepoint, which often just refers to tent stitch. It is also known as tapestry which is really a woven technique.

The range of work it is possible to do varies according to the complexity of the design, the number and variety of stitches, the scale and type of canvas and the colour and kind of yarns used.

Bearing in mind these things, the working of canvas embroidery can be enjoyed by anyone handicapped for example by a lack of mobility, unsteady hands, failing or deteriorating eyesight, lack of grip or by only having the use of one hand.

MATERIALS

Canvas

There are basically two types of embroidery canvas, single or double thread. Single thread canvas is measured by the number of threads to 1in (25mm), and is the most useful when working a wide range of stitches. Double thread canvas is measured by the number of holes to 1in (25mm) and is used for greater firmness when working in cross stitch or its variations.

Canvas is sold in various sizes of mesh and in various widths. The 10 threads per 1in (25mm) size is ideal for most medium weight work such as bags, cushions etc. Rug canvas usually consists of double threads twisted to resemble a single thread canvas, varying from three to five holes per 1in (25mm). Generally the large-scale canvas is easier for those with bad eyesight or unsteady hands.

There is also a kind of plastic canvas which is sold in shapes or in sheets which can be cut to size. This is extremely rigid and will not pull out of shape however much a lack of feeling in the fingers may incline the worker to pull the thread too hard.

Needles

Any needle used must have a rounded end and not a point, which would split the thread. The needle should have an eye large enough for the thread but not large enough to distort the canvas.

Tapestry needles are made specifically for the purpose. Large sacking needles with the point filed to a rounded end are very useful with rug canvas. A needle of this size is easy to grasp for those with little feeling or strength in the fingers and when placed in the correct hole in the canvas will drop through under its own weight.

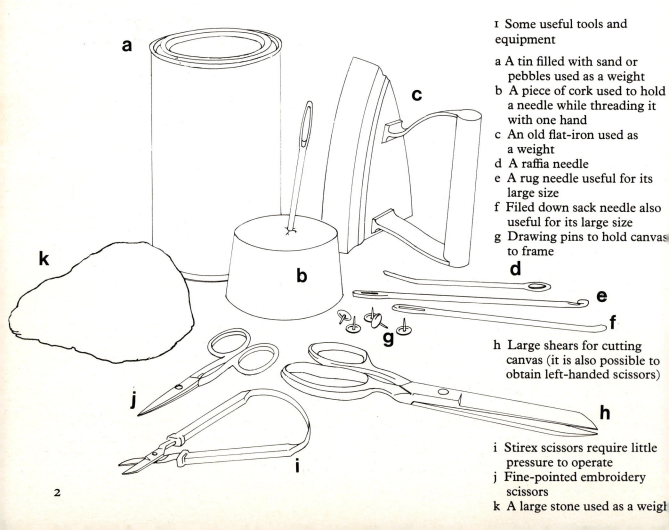

1 Some useful tools and equipment

a A tin filled with sand or pebbles used as a weight
b A piece of cork used to hold a needle while threading it with one hand
c An old flat-iron used as a weight
d A raffia needle
e A rug needle useful for its large size
f Filed down sack needle also useful for its large size
g Drawing pins to hold canvas to frame
h Large shears for cutting canvas (it is also possible to obtain left-handed scissors)
i Stirex scissors require little pressure to operate
j Fine-pointed embroidery scissors
k A large stone used as a weight

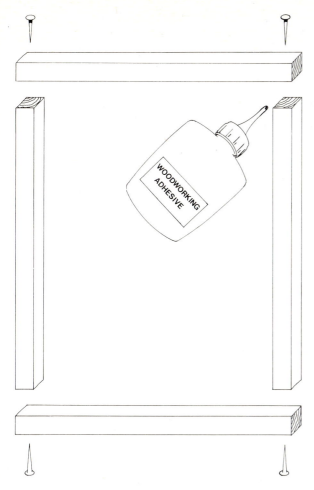

2 Constructing a frame

Frames

Frames are sometimes useful for working with light weight canvas to hold the work in shape and to keep it rigid while in progress. The frame must be rectangular; a circular frame would distort the canvas. There are a range of commercially available frames, some on stands, some with movable sides and others with rotating ends. A particularly useful type is one which rotates on a central axis but locks into position. It is therefore easy for someone with limited use of the hands or the use of one hand only, to turn the work over to fasten off ends on the back. However it is possible to use an old wooden picture frame or to make a simple frame yourself (*fig 2*). If you prefer not to use a frame and the work does pull out of shape you can damp stretch the work afterwards (see p 16).

Yarns

A yarn used for embroidery should be colour fast and thick enough to cover the canvas with no gaps or canvas threads showing. One or more strands can be used and may vary according to the stitch used.

Tapestry wool is available in a wide range of shaded colours but unfortunately it is expensive. *Knitting yarns* of various kinds are quite satisfactory. *Carpet thrums* (ends of wool left over in carpet production) are sometimes available from carpet manufacturers and are very strong and durable. *Six ply rug wool* is usually sold for making tufted rugs but can also be used for embroidery. *Plastic raffia*, available in a good range of colours, either matt or lustre finish, gives a bright sheen and is often used in conjunction with other yarns. Nylon strips known as *Nytrim* are washable, can be bought cheaply and may be used with rug canvas.

HOW TO EMBROIDER FOURTEEN DIFFERENT STITCHES

There are a wide range of stitches that can be used in canvas work, most are suitable for use on all types and scales of canvas. There are many comprehensive books on stitches which can be consulted as one becomes more interested and involved in the work. Here are a few that can be tried in a variation of colours and threads. It is often a good idea to start by making an item that contains many stitches, a 'sampler'; this can be a bag, cushion or small rug. In this way you can find out which stitches you like and are able to manage best.

Florentine stitch *(fig 3)*

Also known as bargello or flame stitch, this is a straight stitch worked parallel over the same number of threads, most commonly over four threads, but it can vary from two to eight.

Hungarian stitch *(fig 4)*

This stitch is made up of groups of three, two short stitches and a long one. Two threads must be left between each group to allow the next row to fit in.

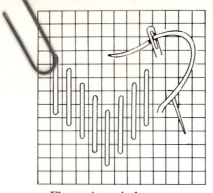

3 Florentine stitch

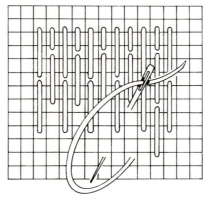

4 Hungarian stitch

5a Brick stitch

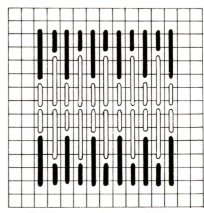

5b Variation on long and short stitch

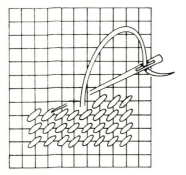

6a Tent stitch, worked in a straight line

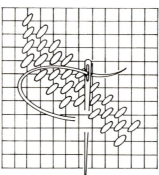

6b Tent stitch, worked on the diagonal

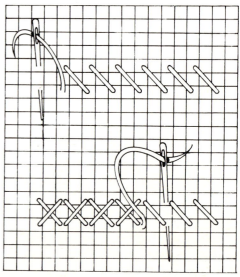

7 Cross stitch

Brick stitch (fig 5a)

The first row must be worked with a long and a short stitch over two and four threads respectively. The following rows are over four threads with a step down of two thus giving a brick formation. A variation on the long and short stitch can be worked in rows (fig 5b).

Tent stitch (fig 6a)

Also known as petit point or basket weave when worked diagonally, tent stitch is usually worked on single thread canvas in rows. It has a tendency to pull the canvas so it is helpful to use a frame. When tent stitch is worked diagonally (fig 6b) a strong woven texture is formed on the reverse of the work hence the name basket weave; is suitable for rugs as it is hard-wearing.

Cross stitch (fig 7)

Work a row of slanting stitches, then work back over the first row in the opposite direction to form the cross. This is a good way of ensuring that all the crosses lie in the same direction.

Double cross stitch (fig 8)

A cross stitch is worked first then another cross stitch worked over the top, set at a diagonal to the first cross. Interesting effects can be created with the use of two colours, one for the cross underneath and a contrasting colour for the cross on top.

Sheaf stitch (fig 9)

This stitch, as the name suggests, resembles a sheaf of corn. It consists of working three vertical stitches over four threads then tying round the middle with two stitches.

Rice stitch (fig 10)

First work a row of cross stitch over at least two threads either way, as in a double cross stitch, then work small stitches across the corners of the large cross. This stitch is also ideal for working in two colours.

Star stitch (fig 11a)

Star stitch consists of straight stitches worked into a central hole; care must be taken that the canvas does not show through. Sometimes a long stitch must be worked in between the star stitch to cover any gaps (fig 11b).

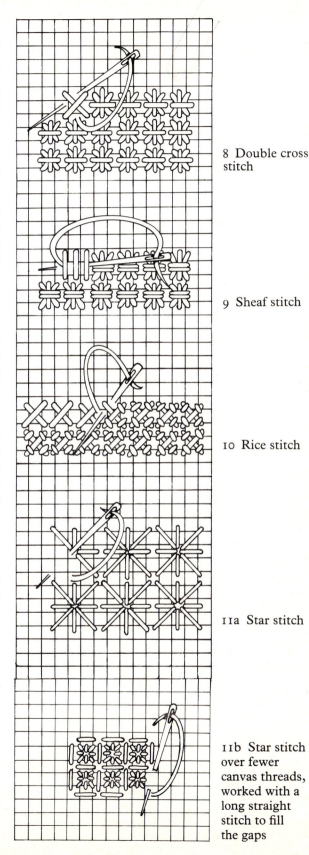

8 Double cross stitch

9 Sheaf stitch

10 Rice stitch

11a Star stitch

11b Star stitch over fewer canvas threads, worked with a long straight stitch to fill the gaps

5

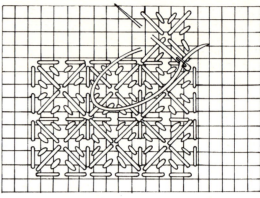

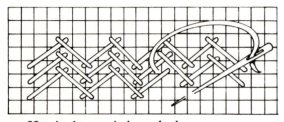

12 Herringbone stitch worked
over two threads in each
direction

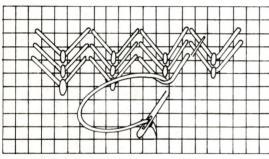

13 Fly stitch

14 Double star stitch

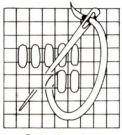

15 Gobelin stitch

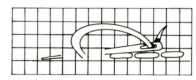

16 Back stitch

Herringbone stitch *(fig 12)*
When working herringbone stitch on canvas it
is important to experiment with the number of
threads worked over to ensure that the canvas is
covered. The second row is worked one thread
down from the first, so that the rows interlock
closely.

Fly stitch *(fig 13)*
This is also known as Y stitch. Although not
traditionally a canvas stitch it can be worked on
canvas with pleasing results either in rows
horizontally or vertically. The effect is almost
like knitting when worked on canvas. It is a
straight stitch pulled into a V-shape and tied
down with another stitch which can vary in
length. When used as a canvas stitch the tying-
down stitch should be over not more than two
threads. When worked horizontally the rows
interlock in a similar way to herringbone.

Double star stitch *(fig 14)*
This stitch is worked over a square of four
threads. The long diagonal stitches from the
corners to the centre hole are worked first,
smaller stitches that form a V-shape are worked
in the four spaces, leaving the middle holes of
the four edges free for the four large stitches
into the centre hole. Straight stitches over two
threads are then worked round the whole of the
square.

Gobelin stitch *(fig 15)*
This stitch is worked vertically in straight
rows. It can be worked in different lengths.

Back stitch *(fig 16)*
This stitch is generally used to stitch fabrics
but is often useful to fill in gaps in canvas
embroidery where the canvas shows.

IDEAS ON WHAT TO MAKE

Game boards
Picture frame
Cushion
Pin cushion
Needle case
Belt
Waistcoat
Trimmings for garments
Purse
Slippers
Bag
Pencil case
Book cover
Spectacle case
Picture or wall hanging
Bathroom scales
Rug
Chair seats
Stool top
Table mats

CHOOSING A DESIGN

Colour

People often think that there is something mysterious about choosing the right colour, but in nature the most unlikely, vibrant colours are next to each other without looking wrong. Colour is very personal and what is pleasing to one person is not necessarily so to another. Superstition about colour is quite common; 'blue and green should never be seen' is one of many old wives' tales. Manufacturers create fashions in certain colours in order to increase sales. This year's new colour was probably new five years ago under a different name.

Start by looking around at colour; it is everywhere, and you may be surprised at the combinations that you find. In your use of colours make sure that you like them as you may become discouraged if you are unhappy about the colours you are working with. Some combinations of colours can be disturbing to some people and literally make them feel ill.

A wallpaper sample book will often help you to decide what colours you like and dislike as they often have the same pattern in various colourways. With careful positioning of a few colours you can create the effect of many more than are actually used; each colour affects its neighbour. It can also be helpful to try your coloured yarns against each other in various combinations to give you an idea of possible effects. If you are making furnishings of some kind the colours should blend with the decor.

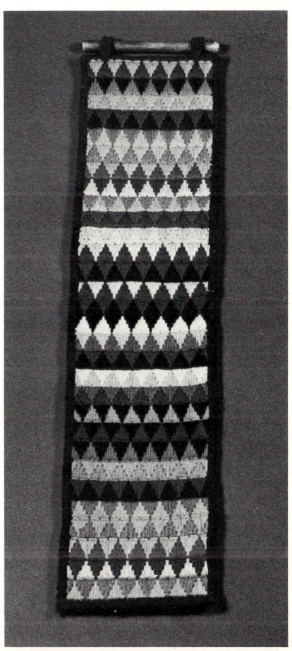

17 Examples of articles made with canvas embroidery (continued over)

7

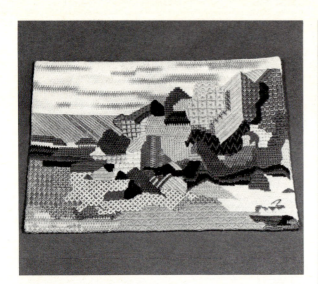

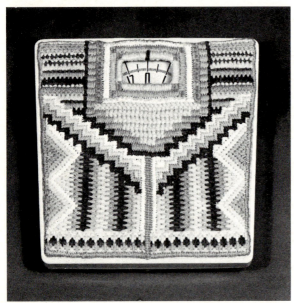

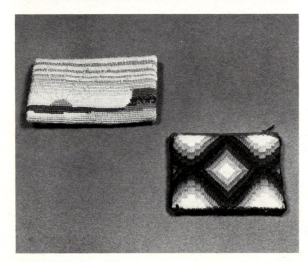

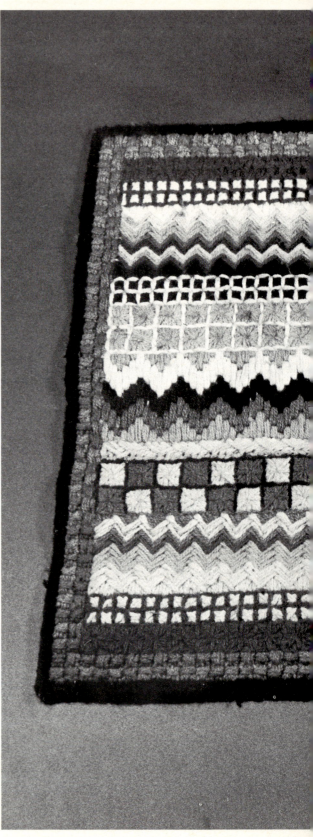

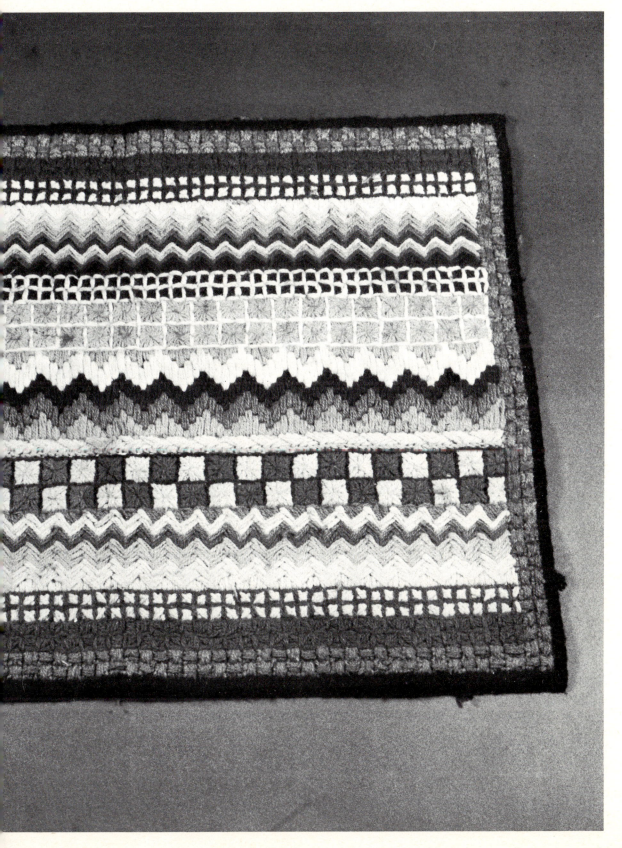

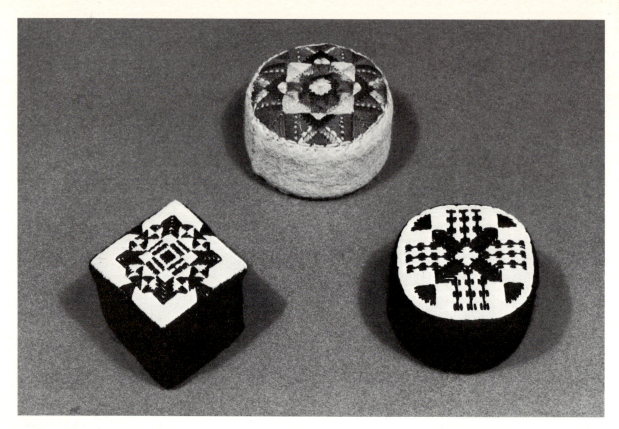

17 (continued) Examples of
articles made with canvas embroidery

PUTTING YOUR DESIGN INTO PRACTICE

Stitches

If you are making an article of use rather than something to hang on the wall make sure none of the stitches you choose have long floating threads as these will catch and spoil the work.

Shape

The finished article need not be rectangular or square. A bag for instance could be made up in many ways: do you want it to have a gusset, will it have a front flap, how will it be fastened if at all, what kind of handle will it have?

Pattern

People with eyesight difficulties may find some types of pattern hard to work on. Particularly vivid patterning such as some stripes or zigzag patterns may be disturbing to some people.

Scale

The scale of the work can be quite varied but generally the larger the scale the easier it is to work on.

A design can come from many sources: from nature, pictures, photographs, or a pattern can be adapted from one in use, for example on a piece of fabric or wallpaper. An idea may begin with a shape you like, an arrangement of colours, a stitch you want to try out or a need for a particular article.

There are three ways of setting about designing a piece of canvas embroidery:
• Graph paper, because of its squared format, is ideal for canvas designs. Each square can be used to represent one hole of the canvas, or one stitch. The design can be worked onto the graph paper using felt-tip pens and then used as a pattern to follow square by square when working on the canvas (fig 18).
• The design can be drawn on paper first then the canvas placed over it and the design traced directly onto the canvas.
• With less complex patterns the threads can be worked directly onto the canvas, stitches and colours being worked out as you go.

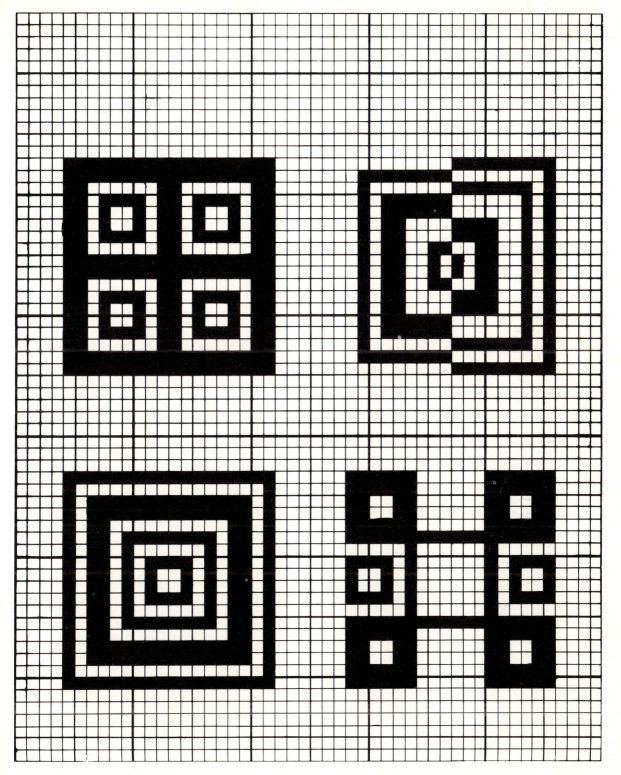

18 Designs drawn on graph paper (continued over)

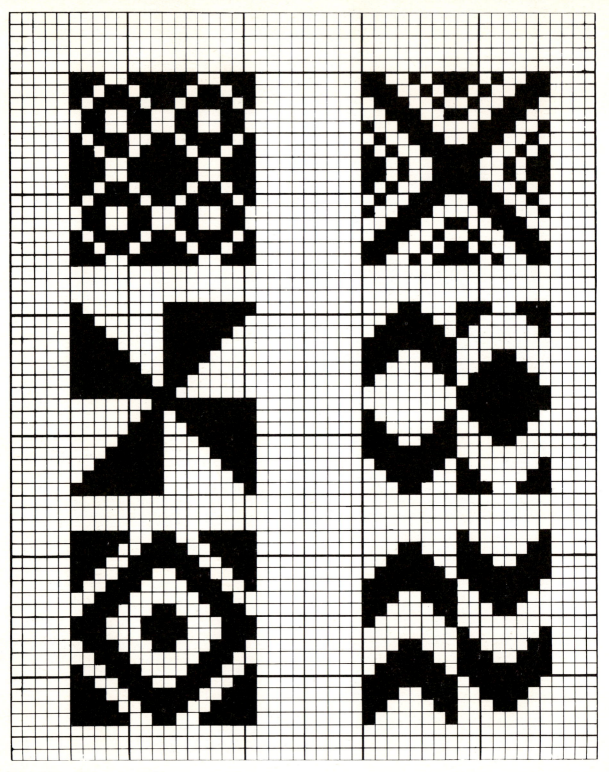

18 Designs drawn on graph
paper (continued)

12

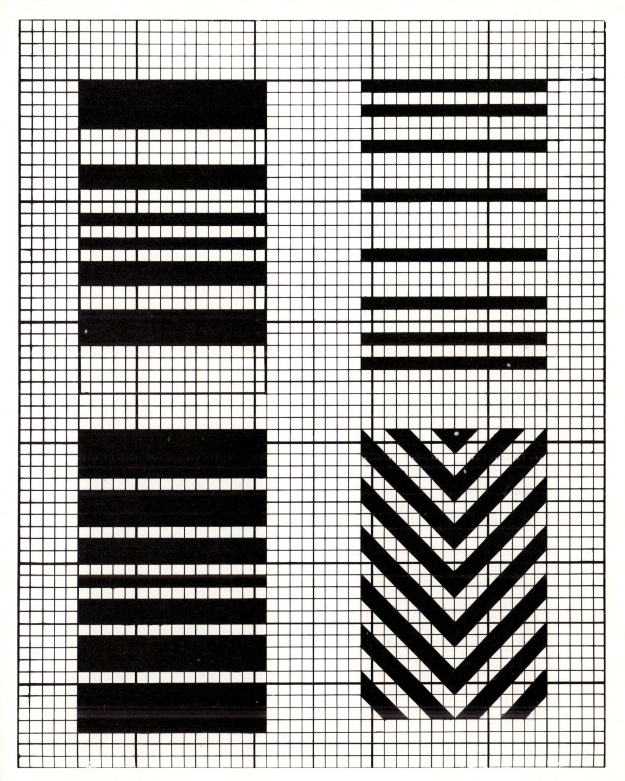

18 Designs drawn on graph
paper (continued)

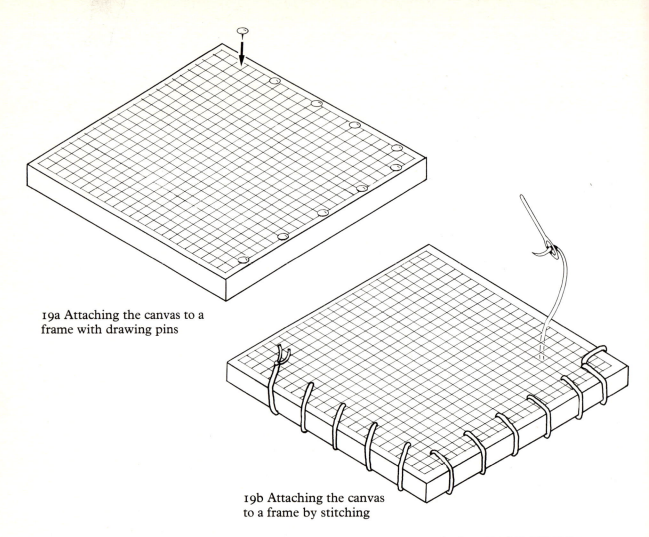

19a Attaching the canvas to a
frame with drawing pins

19b Attaching the canvas
to a frame by stitching

HINTS ON WORKING

Canvas can be attached to a frame by one of two methods. It can be quite simply pinned on using drawing pins (*fig 19a*). Alternatively it can be stitched on using a strong thread (*fig 19b*).

It is a good idea to oversew the raw edges of your canvas to stop it fraying while you are working (*fig 20*).

When you begin work, have a knot in your thread on the right side, a short distance away from where you are actually going to start stitching. A thread will lie across the back for this short distance which you work over. When you reach the knot cut it off (*fig 21*).

If you work the stitches in two movements, once bringing the needle up through the canvas and once down, it will help to keep the canvas in

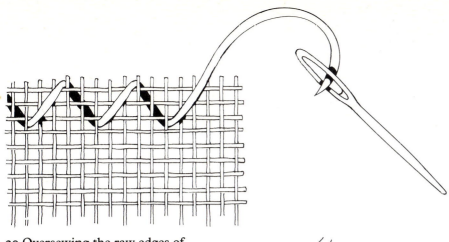

20 Oversewing the raw edges of
the canvas

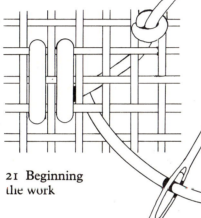

21 Beginning
the work

shape and the stitches even.

Once the work is begun and you are sometimes working into a hole in the canvas that
has a thread already in it, make sure that you
work downwards into that hole so that any
splitting of threads that may occur will happen
on the back of your work.

If you are inclined to drop the needle
occasionally while working and you are using
double threads, thread it with a loop through
the needle (*fig 22*).

When using plastic canvas with a large
tapestry needle and a fine thread like raffia, it is
possible to knot the thread onto the needle (*fig
23*).

It is often helpful to use a weight of some
kind to hold the work still (*fig 1, p 2*).

To finish off a piece of thread run it along the
stitches on the back of the work. After the first
time you can start a new thread in the same way.

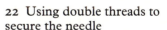
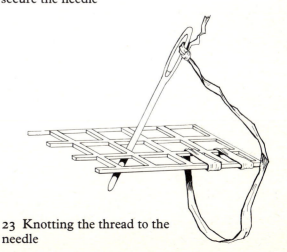

22 Using double threads to
secure the needle

23 Knotting the thread to the
needle

MAKING UP AND FINISHING

Damp stretching

When a piece of canvas has been pulled out of shape through working on it, as quite often happens with tent stitch, it needs to be damp stretched. This is quite a simple operation for which you will need a flat board larger than the piece to be stretched, drawing pins, a couple of large sheets of absorbent paper and a cup of water.

Pin a sheet of paper to the board so that one edge of the paper is level with one edge of the board, then draw a line parallel with this edge, 2 in (50 mm) from it. Use drawing pins to hold one of the edges of the piece of work along this line (this edge is the end of the line of stitching not the edge of the canvas), (fig 24). Then pin the opposite edge, pulling the work into shape as necessary. Continue pinning all sides of the piece of work until the canvas is the shape you require. The drawing pins should be at intervals of 1 in (25 mm) or even closer together depending on how out of shape the canvas is.

Now sprinkle water over the stitched area so that it becomes damp, not soaking wet. Cover with another sheet of paper and leave to dry for a couple of days or however long it takes. Then remove paper and pins and your piece of work should remain in the shape you pinned it to.

Backing

A piece of canvas embroidery that is to be used flat, such as a rug, wall hanging or table mat, may require backing, especially if the work is not very neat on the back. Hessian is very suitable for backing a rug or hanging. Cut the hessian slightly larger than the work. Hem it securely to the back of the work using a strong thread in self colour, turning under the raw edges of the hessian so that it is slightly smaller than the finished size of the rug (fig 25).

With smaller items, such as table mats, felt is very useful. You can choose from a wide range of colours to match your work. Cut the felt slightly smaller than the mat and glue onto the back using a rubber-based glue such as Copydex. This type of glue remains flexible after it has dried so there is no risk of the glue cracking and the backing coming away.

To make a twisted cord

Cut several lengths of wool three times as long as the required finished length of the cord. Put a knot at each end and attach one end to a door knob and holding the other end, move far enough away so that the threads are taut.

Put a pencil in front of the knot and holding the threads just in front of the pencil with the left hand, with the right hand keeep turning the pencil clockwise until the threads are tightly twisted (fig 26).

Fold the cord in half, placing the knotted ends together, still keeping the threads taut. Gradually release from the fold end a few inches at a time and the threads will all twist together forming the cord. Knot all the ends together and trim off your original knots.

It is quicker to make the cord if there are two people, one at either end, with both of them twisting at the same time in opposite directions from each other.

Alternatively you could make a braid by plaiting strands of the wools used.

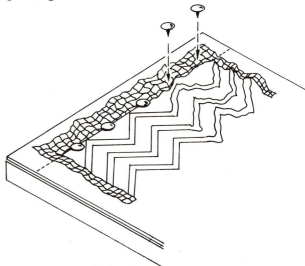

24 Damp stretching with edge of stitching pinned along drawn line, parallel with edge of board

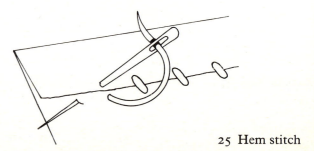

25 Hem stitch

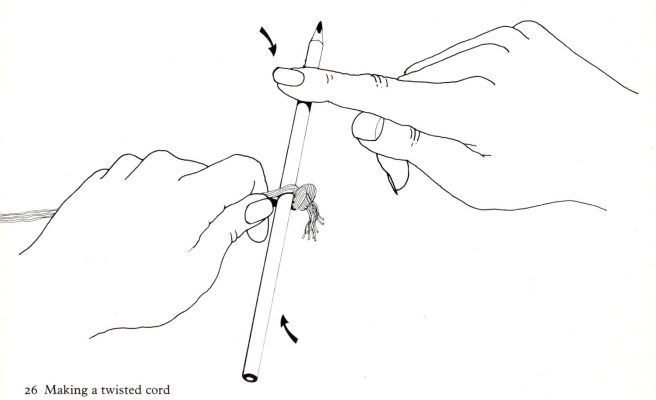

26 Making a twisted cord

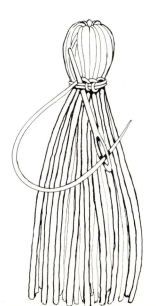

27 Buttonhole stitch on a tassel

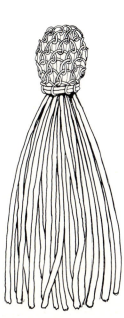

28 Finished buttonholing on a tassel

To make a fancy tassel

Knot together a good-sized bunch of threads and fold them down over the knot. Thread a tapestry needle with wool and secure it to the knot. Wind the thread in the needle twice round the tassel just below the knot, but not too tightly. Work around these two threads in buttonhole stitch (*fig 27*). On the second and subsequent rows work into the top of each stitch on the previous row, continuing upwards. Pull the last two rows in tightly to follow the shape of the top of the tassel (*fig 28*). Fasten off.

To hang a picture or wall hanging

You need a piece of bamboo or dowelling rod (obtainable from DIY shops) slightly wider than the finished width of the embroidery. The backing fabric needs to be a few inches longer than usual. Stitch the backing fabric along the sides and base of the work with the long end at the top, take this over in a loop and back into itself (*fig 29a*). Stitch securely along level with the top of the embroidery. Run the bamboo or

17

dowelling into the loop (*fig 29b*).

An alternative method would be to have several narrow loops rather than one long one, attached to the top of the work (*fig 29c*).

Fringing

A piece of work can be fringed using this simple method. Cut fringes twice the finished length plus 1in (25mm). Insert a crochet hook into the work upwards and lay a loop of the fringe over the hook. Pull the loop through the canvas, thread the two ends through and pull tight (*fig 30*). Repeat along the edge.

Making up a cushion

If you do not have a cushion ready for an embroidered cover, it is easy to make one. You need two pieces of calico or sheeting, cut to the shape and size you require. Machine or back stitch round the edges leaving a hand's width open. Turn through and stuff firmly with whatever stuffing you are using (see chapter 2, Soft Toys, p 30). Ladder stitch the open edges together (*fig 31*).

A fabric for backing a cushion needs to be firm and hard-wearing such as hessian or corduroy. Cut the backing fabric the same size as the canvas. Pin the canvas and backing right sides together with the pins across the stitching line instead of with it. It can then be machined or back stitched round over the pins, stitching three sides and working from the canvas side (*figs 32a, 32b*). Trim the edges, cutting across the corners, and turn through to the right side. Slip the cushion inside the cover and ladder stitch along the edges of the open side. If the canvas threads show along the seam you may like to put a cord or braid round the edges.

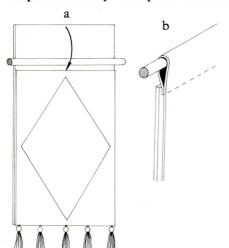

29 Methods of hanging

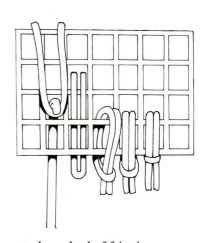

30 A method of fringing

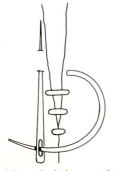

31 Ladder stitch is a method of joining two edges together invisibly; it is worked by taking small stitches alternately into each edge

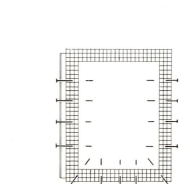

32a Pinning the finished embroidery to the backing

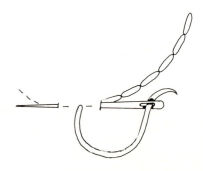

32b Back stitch on fabric

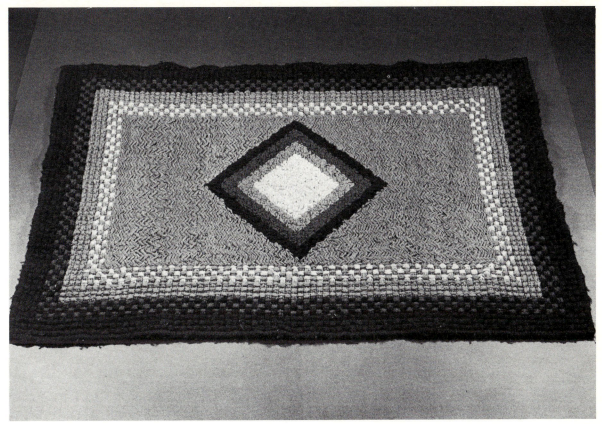

33 Rug

RUG

This rug measures approximately 36in × 53in (92cm × 135cm) when completed – a convenient size for either a hearth or bedside rug. As it is made using 6-ply wool it is also fairly hard-wearing.

Materials

Single mesh rug canvas
18 skeins of 6-ply rug wool, with the following number of skeins in each colour (using Melrose rug wool colours): 2 Spanish Yellow, 2 Old Gold, 2 Dark Amber, 4 Tobacco Brown, 2 Teal Blue, 6 Aqua (figs 34a, 34b).

Instructions

It is best to work the edging first as it helps to keep the canvas in shape and stop the ends from fraying (fig 35).

Work simple edging over the selvedge; it may be necessary to turn one of the selvedges under. The raw edges should be turned under by five threads and worked on double. The required number of threads to work the pattern are 118 threads wide by 178 threads long, so turn under accordingly. The corners are worked by going into the same hole several times and spreading the wool evenly round the corner (fig 36).

The border is worked in double cross stitch in a chequered design of browns and blues lightening in tone towards the centre.

Next work the central diamond starting from the middle hole, which is the centre of the first star stitch. An extra straight stitch will be needed along each side of the star stitch to cover any gaps showing in the canvas (fig 37).

The remaining canvas is filled in with herringbone stitch worked over two threads in either direction (fig 12, p6). Run all ends into the back of the other stitches while working; if this is done neatly it is not necessary to put any backing on the rug.

Design chart (worked in double cross stitch). The grid is a letter-coded color chart forming an L-shaped rug border.

Top (wide) block:

```
E N E N E N E N E N E N E N E N E N E N E N
N E N E N E N E N E N E N E N E N E N E N E
E N E N E N E N E N E N E N E N E N E N E N
N E N E H E H E H E H E H E H E H E H E H E
E N E H E H E H E H E H E H E H E H E H E H
N E N E H E H E H E H E H E H E H E H E H E
E N E H E H O T O T O T O T O T O T O T O T
N E N E H E T O T O T O T O T O T O T O T O
E N E H E H O T O T O T O T O T O T O T O T
N E N E H E T O T O S O S O S O S O S O S O
E N E H E H O T O S O S O S O S O S O S O S
N E N E H E T O T O S O S O S O S O S O S O
```

Lower (narrow) block:

```
E N E H E H O T O S O S
N E N E H E T O T O S O
E N E H E H O T O S O S
N E N E H E T O T O S O
E N E H E H O T O S O S
N E N E H E T O T O S O
E N E H E H O T O S O S
N E N E H E T O T O S O
E N E H E H O T O S O S
N E N E H E T O T O S O
E N E H E H O T O S O S
N E N E H E T O T O S O
E N E H E H O T O S O S
N E N E H E T O T O S O
E N E H E H O T O S O S
N E N E H E T O T O S O
E N E H E H O T O S O S
N E N E H E T O T O S O
E N E H E H O T O S O S
N E N E H E T O T O S O
E N E H E H O T O S O S
N E N E H E T O T O S O
E N E H E H O T O S O S
N E N E H E T O T O S O
E N E H E H O T O S O S
N E N E H E T O T O S O
```

Legend:

- **E** Teal brown
- **H** Dark amber
- **S** Spanish yellow
- **O** Aqua
- **T** Old gold
- **N** Tobacco brown

34a Design for border of rug worked in double cross stitch

O Tobacco brown
E Spanish yellow
U Old gold
N Dark amber

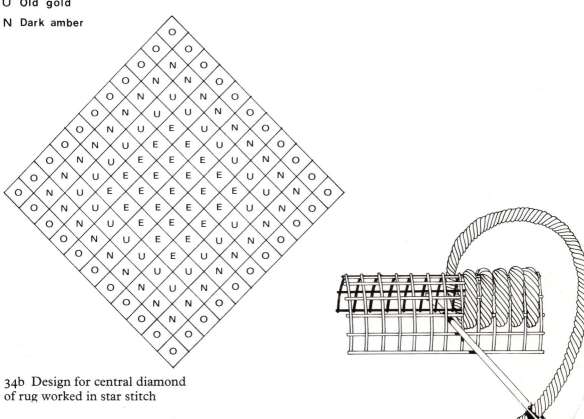

34b Design for central diamond
of rug worked in star stitch

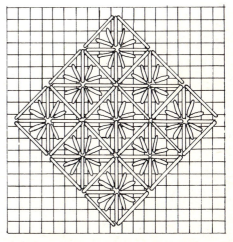

35 Method of working rug
edging with raw canvas folded
over

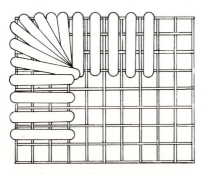

36 Corner of rug edge with
several stitches worked in the
same hole and spread round the
corner

37 Star stitch with long straight
stitch filling gaps

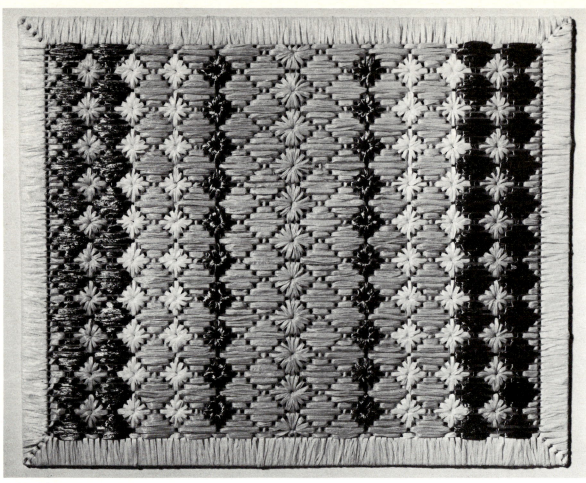

38 Table mat

TABLE MAT

Materials
Plastic canvas mat
2 skeins each of 4 colours imitation raffia
Piece of matching felt 11 in × 14 in (27 cm × 35 cm)
Tapestry needle

Instructions
Using colour A oversew round the edge, sewing over the first five threads of the canvas. Try to spread out the raffia flat so that it covers the plastic completely. Work the corners (fig 40).

1st row, colour B: Start in the centre of the row on the narrow edge of the mat. The stitch used is Hungarian stitch worked over 1, 3, 5, 7 threads. You will have an incomplete stitch at each end of the row.

2nd row, colour C: Work in star stitch to fit into the spaces left by the previous row.

3rd row, colour B: Hungarian stitch
4th row, colour A: Star stitch
5th row, colour C: Hungarian stitch
6th row, colour A: Star stitch
7th row, colour C: Hungarian stitch
8th row, colour B: Star stitch
9th row, colour D: Hungarian stitch
10th row, colour C: Hungarian stitch

Repeat these colours and stitches in this order from the other end.

Fill in the central row with an elongated star stitch in colour D.

Fill in the gaps at each end left by the first row with colour D (fig 41).

Use a latex-based glue such as Copydex to glue the felt onto the back of the work.

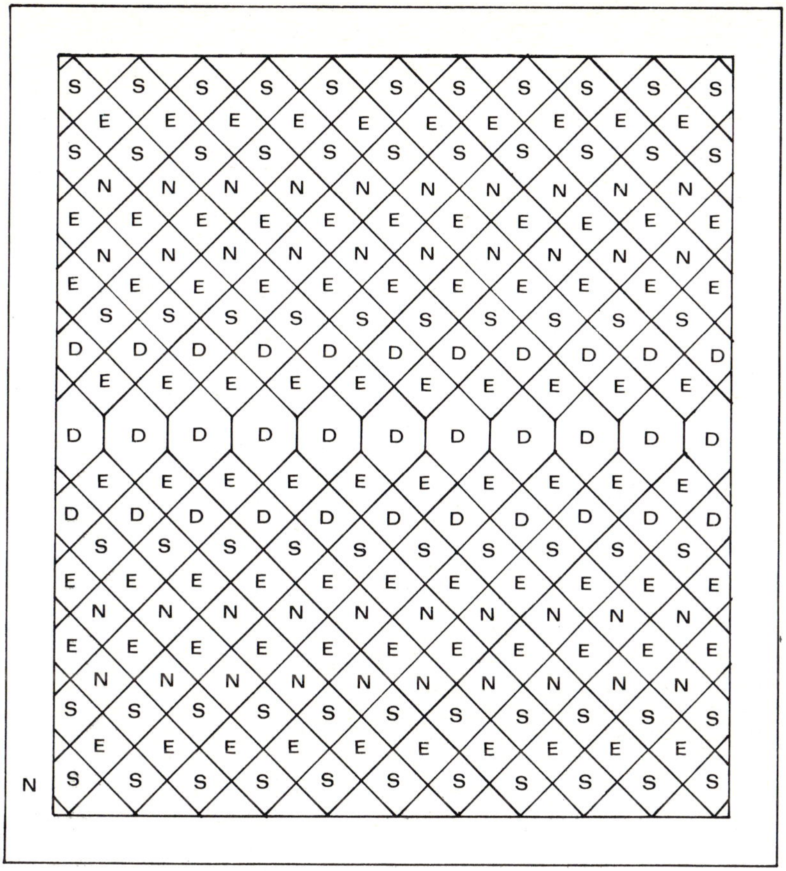
S S S S S S S S S S S
E E E E E E E E E E
S S S S S S S S S S S
N N N N N N N N N N
E E E E E E E E E E E
N N N N N N N N N N
E E E E E E E E E E E
S S S S S S S S S S
D D D D D D D D D D D
E E E E E E E E E E
D D D D D D D D D D D
E E E E E E E E E E
D D D D D D D D D D D
S S S S S S S S S S
E E E E E E E E E E E
N N N N N N N N N N
E E E E E E E E E E E
N N N N N N N N N N
S S S S S S S S S S S
E E E E E E E E E E
S S S S S S S S S S S
N

39 Design for plastic canvas mat worked in star stitch and Hungarian stitch

S Brown

E Orange

N Yellow

D Beige

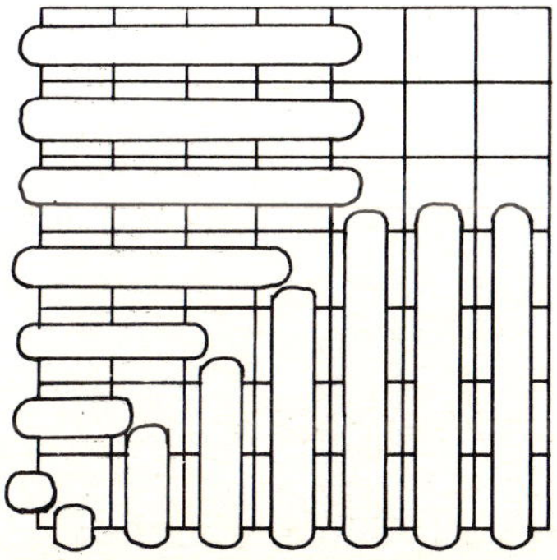

40 Working the corners

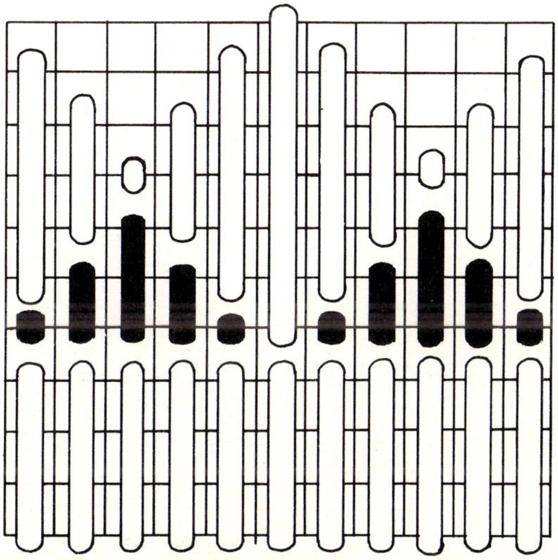

41 Filling in the last spaces

SMALL SHOULDER BAG

Materials
Single thread canvas (10 holes per inch (25mm)), 12in × 10in (30cm × 25cm)
Red needlecord, 12in × 10in (30cm × 25cm)
Dark brown lining, 12in × 20in (30cm × 50cm)
Double knitting wool, 10 × 1 oz (or 20g) balls, 5 shades each of 2 basic colours (eg, 5 shades of red from pale pink to maroon and 5 shades of brown from cream to dark brown) (fig 43)
A frame if you wish to use one

Instructions
Find the centre of the canvas and begin at the base point. Using two threads together, work the five triangles in Hungarian stitch. The bottom point of the second triangle will come to the centre of the top row of the first.

The parallelogram shapes on each side of the top four triangles are then worked in brick stitch. It is necessary to work diagonally because of the colour arrangement.

The corner triangles either side of the top three parallelograms are also worked in brick stitch. Turn the canvas sideways and work diagonally.

Still with the canvas sideways, work two rows of brick stitch around the bottom point of the bag.

Work two rows of gobelin stitch across the top of the bag.

If the canvas shows at all it may be necessary to run a row of back stitch between the two rows of gobelin stitch and also along the top of each triangle.

Making up
Stitch canvas to needlecord (see instructions for cushion cover on p 18) and turn through to the right side.

Fold the lining in half and tack along the stitching line, which you measure slightly smaller than the bag itself. Machine or back stitch by hand. Put the lining inside the bag, turn ends to the inside and ladder stitch round the top.

Make a twisted cord using five lengths of wool each 3½yds (4m) long. Knot both ends of the finished cord together to make a loop.

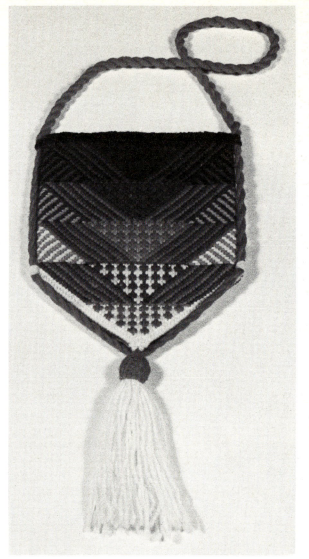

42 Small shoulder bag

Make a tassel using 26 threads each 12in (30cm) long, folding them over the knot in the twisted cord loop. Thread a tapestry needle with wool and secure it to the knot. Wind the thread tightly twice round the cords just above the knot (fig 44). Take the needle and thread through the knot and wind twice round the tassel just below the knot but not too tightly (fig 45). Continue as for tassel instructions on p 17. To finish stitch onto the point at the base of the bag (fig 46).

Finally attach the cord along the sides of the bag by stitching through the bag and over the cord several times, at the top and the bottom of each side (fig 47).

43 Design for shoulder bag

A	Pale pink	1	Cream
B	Pink	2	Beige
C	Rose	3	Tan
D	Red	4	Brown
E	Maroon	5	Dark brown

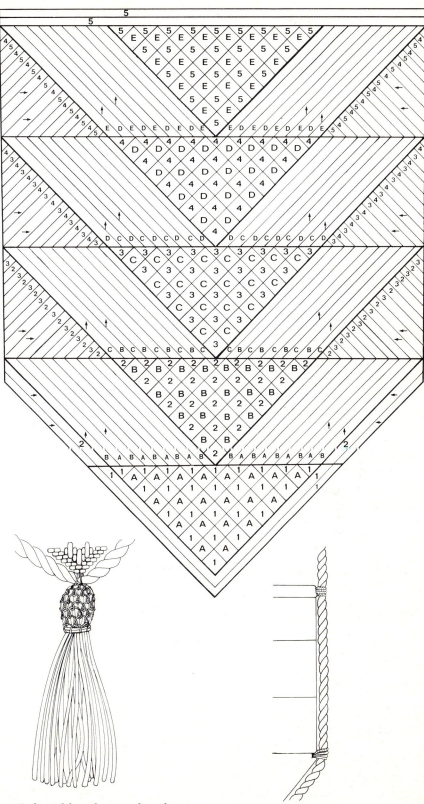

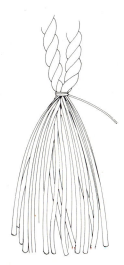

44 Attaching the wool for the tassel to the cord

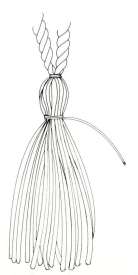

45 Winding the threads to start the buttonhole stitch

46 Attaching the tassel to the bag

47 Attaching the cord to the bag

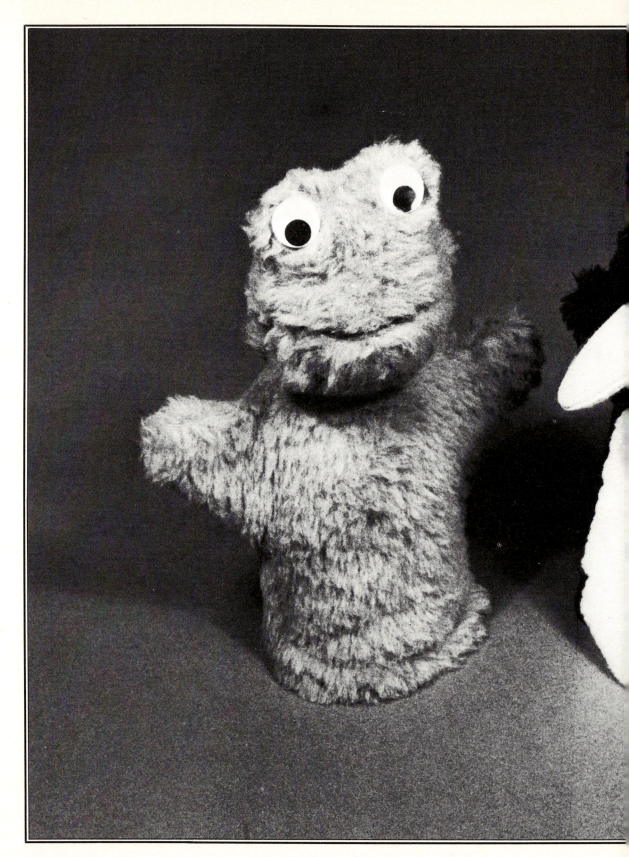

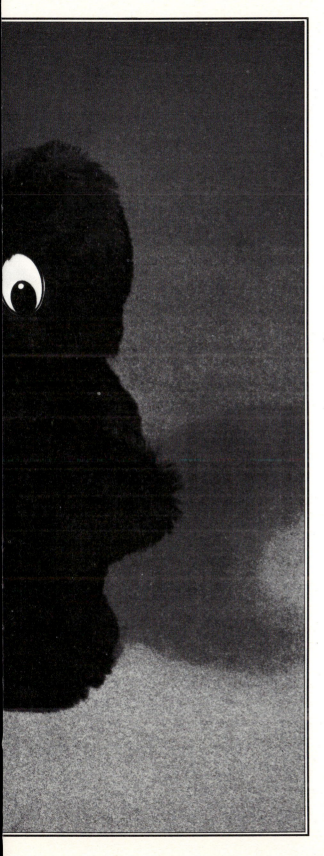

2 Soft Toys

Soft toys offer a tremendous variety, appealing to people of all ages. The work is light to hold and can be very simple to do. Scraps of fabric can be used, so that toy making is very economical, and the use of fur fabric goes a long way to hide uneven stitching (without sacrificing strength). As sewing is usually done fairly close to the edge, people with limited sight can sew using the edge of the fabric as a guide. One-handed workers can use weights to help cutting out and a vice to hold the work while stitching.

As soft toys are usually for children, safety is a very important consideration. Any materials used should not be inflammable. This can easily be tested by setting light to a small piece. It is very important that there are no pins left in the work; they can easily be lost in fur fabric. All features that are attached separately, such as eyes or ears on toy animals, should be very firm so they cannot be pulled off and swallowed.

TOOLS AND EQUIPMENT

Sewing needles

These can be of a more substantial size than usual if that makes them easier to handle and a large eye makes threading easier. It is also possible to buy self-threading needles (*fig 1c*). It is often helpful to use a double thread knotted together if the needle comes unthreaded easily (*fig 22, p 15*). A bodkin or large tapestry needle is useful for threading elastic.

Needle threaders

Small plastic machines are available in which the needle is placed, the thread laid across and a lever pressed to put the thread through the eye (*fig 1i*). It can also be useful to have a piece of cork or a pincushion to hold the needle while it is being threaded (*fig 1, p 2*).

Scissors

Stirex scissors require very little pressure to work and are much less tiring on the hands. People with arthritic hands will often find these scissors very useful. Otherwise a pair of cutting-out shears (right- or left-handed to suit) and a pair of small pointed embroidery scissors will be needed (*figs 1m, 1j and 1n*).

Toy maker's needle

This long needle, made specially for stitching through a toy without getting lost in the middle, is very useful. Alternatively use a very long darning needle (*figs 1d and 1f*).

Pins

It is best to use coloured glass headed pins which can easily be seen. It is very important not to leave any pins in a toy. It is also useful to have a few extra long pins such as macramé pins, T pins or hat pins to pin ears etc, into position before sewing (*figs 1b and 1e*).

Tailor's chalk and pencil

To mark fabrics use chalk for dark colours, pencil for light colours (*fig 1k*).

Stuffing stick

A stick can be made from a piece of $\frac{3}{4}$ in (27mm) dowelling, sanded down thinner at one end and

rounded off at both ends. Or use a large wooden knitting needle instead (*fig 1o*).

Suede brush

This is useful for brushing fur toys when complete (*fig 1p*).

Non-slip mat

Dycem is the name of a kind of non-slip plastic sheet which can be laid on a work surface, so that paper (also some fabrics), when placed on it for marking or cutting, will not slip away. This is particularly useful for people with the use of one hand only (*fig 1l*).

Weights

Any kinds of weights are useful for one-handed workers to hold fabric in place while marking and cutting out (*fig 1g*).

1 Some useful tools and equipment

a A vice
b Glass-headed pins
c Self-threading needle
d Darning needle
e T pin
f Toymaker's needle is like the darning needle but is 6 in (15 cm) long
g Flat iron used as a weight

h A sewing machin[e]
i Witch needle thre[ader]
j Cutting-out shear[s]
k Tailor's chalk
l Dycem non-slip m[at]
m Stirex scissors
n Small, pointed scissors
o Large wooden knitting needle
p Suede brush

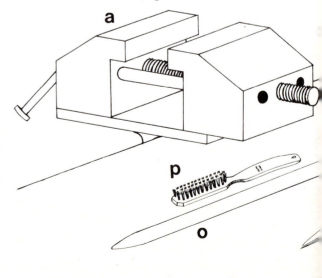

Vice

An ordinary vice clamped to the table can be used to hold work in place while stitching, for people using one hand only. If it is possible, it is sometimes easier to hold the work between the knees (*fig 1a*).

Sewing machines

For those who prefer machining to hand sewing it is possible to adapt many sewing machines to be operated by knee, elbow, chin, mouth etc. Some machines have an automatic needle-threading device or special easy-threading needles (*fig 1h*).

Threads

These must be suitable for the fabric used, ie, synthetic thread for a synthetic fabric. Small amounts of knitting wool are also useful for embroidering features and for doll's hair.

Fabrics

Any fabric for toy making needs to be strong, not too thin or too stretchy. Suitable fabrics are needlecord, hessian, gingham, calico, felt etc. Fur fabric of various kinds is available, usually in 54in (137cm) width, and in a wide range of colours. Fur fabric will tear across the width but not down the length. This is useful when measuring off small amounts at a time from a large bulk of fabric.

Stuffing

There are many kinds of stuffing available, suitable for different purposes.

Kapok is made from natural fibres and although it is very soft and stuffs very evenly it tends to get into the air and would not be suitable for anyone with breathing difficulties or a 'hay fever' type allergy. It is not washable.

Terylene stuffing is available in white (essential for pale coloured toys) or mixed colours. It is harder than Kapok but evenly textured, holds together and is washable. It is suitable for most purposes.

There are various other types of stuffing sold made from fluff collected during the manufacture of some textile goods including fur fabric. These will be terylene, nylon, wool etc, accordingly.

Bags of *foam chips* are also sold for stuffing and are relatively cheap. They are rather hard and give a lumpy uneven feel to a toy. It is better to mix them in with a softer stuffing. This mixture can be an economical stuffing for very large toys.

Odd pieces of fur fabric, soft materials, pairs of old tights (washed) etc, can also be mixed in with a softer stuffing to make a smoother texture than when used on their own.

Transferring patterns

Trace the pattern pieces from the page, marking all the features given. Glue the tracing paper onto card and then cut out the pieces. The patterns can then be used repeatedly without much wear.

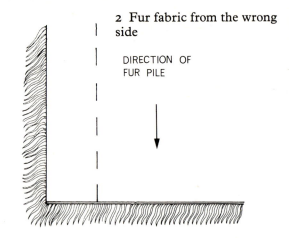

2 Fur fabric from the wrong side

DIRECTION OF FUR PILE

Marking out fur fabric

Lay the fur out with the fur face upwards and run your hand across it to find out the direction in which the pile lies. It is usually parallel with the selvedge. It also helps sometimes to look at the fabric from the wrong side; the pile will protrude at one edge (*fig 2*). Keep the fur face downwards. The pattern pieces are all marked with arrows which must follow the direction of the pile. It is usually more economical to start with the large pieces and try to fit the smaller pieces in between. Draw round the pieces with pencil or tailor's chalk. In most cases where there are two pieces to be marked from the same pattern piece, it is necessary to mark one of them in reverse. First mark in the normal way and then with the pattern piece turned over (still with the arrow pointing in the same direction as the pile). Mark the eye positions and any other features indicated on the pattern.

Cutting out fur fabric

Work from the wrong side of the fur fabric but run the point of the scissors along the pile making a parting so that you only cut the fabric and none of the pile. This is because the fur is directional and straight cutting will leave bald patches along the edges.

Pinning and stitching

To pin fur fabric, place the pieces together, right sides together, and tuck the fur through to the right side as you pin. This helps to make the seams invisible. Oversew all round where you have pinned. The oversewing need not be very close as it is not the main stitching. It acts partly as a tacking stitch and partly helps to strengthen the seam and stop it stretching (*fig 3*). Machine stitch or back stitch just inside the oversewing (*figs 4a, 4b*). Ladder stitch is used to join an opening from the right side eg, after stuffing (*fig 5*). Stab stitch is used where it is necessary for neat stitching to show both sides (*fig 6*). Hem stitch is sometimes used on dolls' clothes (*fig 7*).

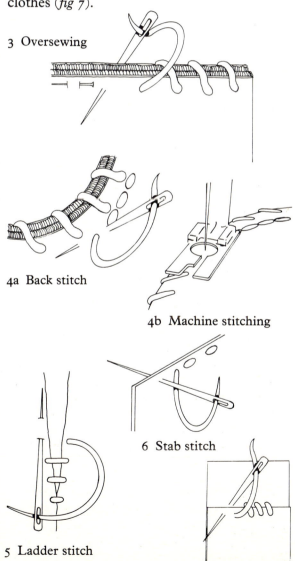

3 Oversewing

4a Back stitch

4b Machine stitching

5 Ladder stitch

6 Stab stitch

7 Hem stitch

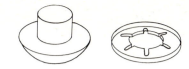

8a Eye with washer

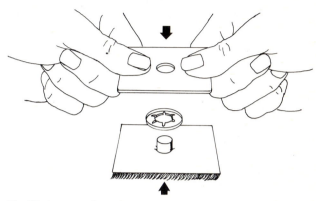

8b Fixing a safety eye

Eyes

Plastic safety eyes have been used for the fur toys but if preferred felt ones can be made and stitched on. Safety eyes in various sizes come in two parts: the eye, which has a shank, and the washer. Some safety eyes need a special tool to fix them, others can be pushed on by hand. First make a hole in the fabric on the marked position using a sharp pointed tool such as a basketry bodkin, a knitting needle or the point of the scissors. Push the shank of the eye through from the right side so that it protrudes through the hole. Push on the washer. For those that require a tool, a small piece of metal with a hole big enough to take the shank of the eye is ideal. It can also be done with a wooden cotton reel and a hammer (*figs 8a, 8b*).

Stuffing

Pull out small pieces of stuffing one at a time and fluff out evenly before putting into the toy. This ensures that the stuffing builds up gradually and evenly until tightly packed with no spaces. If large handfuls are put in at one time the stuffing will be uneven and leave spaces. It can then move about inside the toy which will easily lose its shape. Start with any awkward parts such as pointed noses, arms or legs, pushing each piece of stuffing down firmly with the stuffing stick and work back towards the opening, ensuring that every part is very tightly packed.

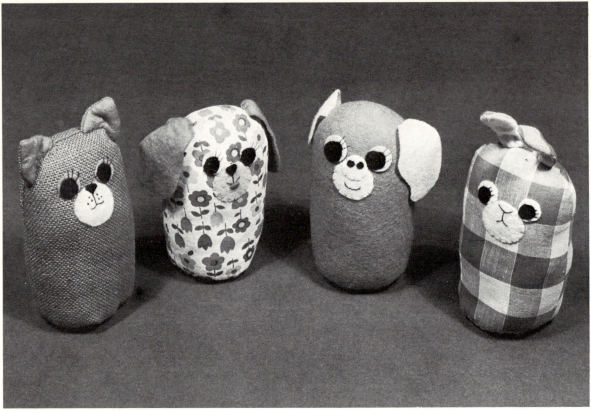

9 Cat, dog, pig, rabbit

ANIMALS FROM SCRAPS OF MATERIAL
CAT · DOG · RABBIT · PIG

Animal toys have a very direct appeal (9). It is quite simple to represent a particular animal without being very realistic. Pick out the most obvious feature of the animal and exaggerate it, rather as a cartoonist might do. With the following animals the characteristic differences are mainly shown by the ears. After you have tried out the patterns given here you may like to design your own animals using the basic body pattern (Pattern 1).

Materials
Piece of fabric, 9in × 14in (23cm × 35cm)
Smaller scraps of the same fabric for ears on rabbit or cat
Pieces of felt for base, ears and features
Matching thread
Black thread for embroidering features
Stuffing

Instructions
Fold the piece of fabric in half so it measures 9in × 7in (23cm × 18cm), with the right side inside. Lay the body pattern on the two layers of fabric and draw round it with a pencil (chalk if the fabric is dark-coloured). Pin the layers together inside the marked line. The drawn line is the stitching line so do not cut out (fig 10).

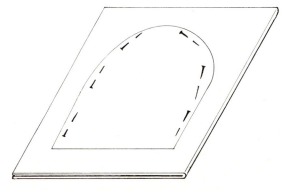

10 Fabric pinned after marking out

PATTERN 1   CAT, DOG, RABBIT and PIG

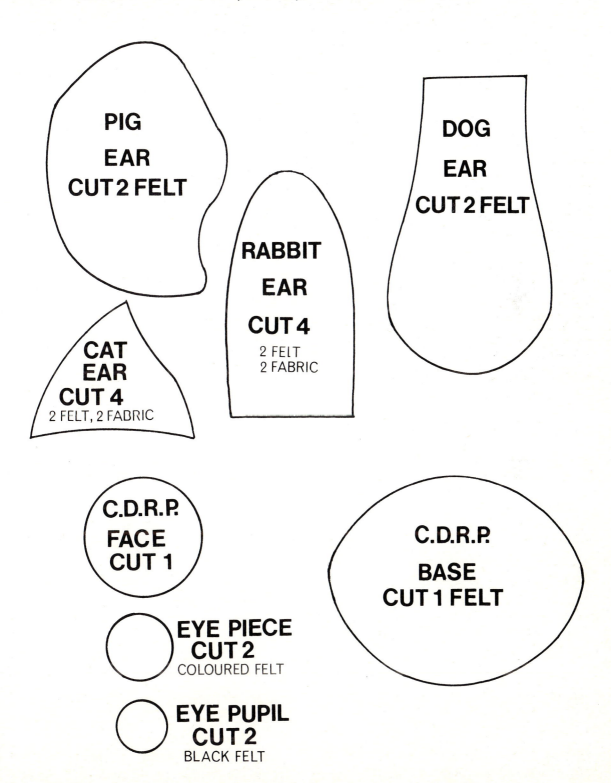

PIG
EAR
CUT 2 FELT

DOG
EAR
CUT 2 FELT

RABBIT
EAR
CUT 4
2 FELT
2 FABRIC

CAT
EAR
CUT 4
2 FELT, 2 FABRIC

C.D.R.P.
FACE
CUT 1

C.D.R.P.
BASE
CUT 1 FELT

EYE PIECE
CUT 2
COLOURED FELT

EYE PUPIL
CUT 2
BLACK FELT

PATTERN 1 CAT, DOG, RABBIT and PIG

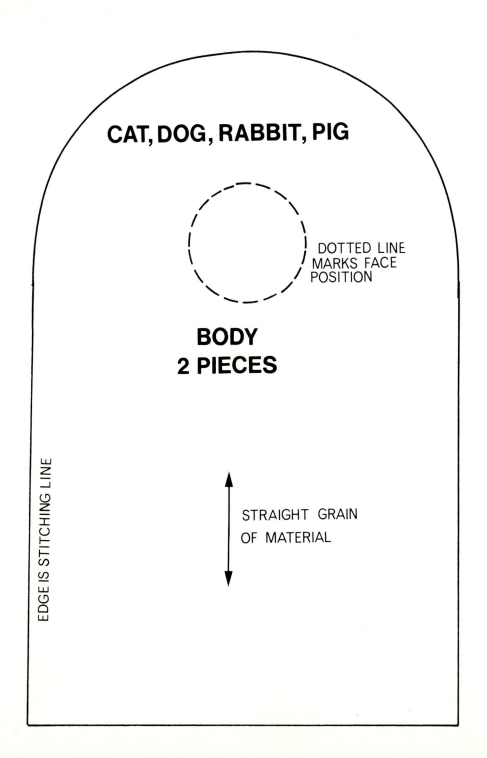

CAT, DOG, RABBIT, PIG

DOTTED LINE
MARKS FACE
POSITION

BODY
2 PIECES

EDGE IS STITCHING LINE

STRAIGHT GRAIN
OF MATERIAL

Mark the felt pieces for the ears (fabric pieces for the cat and rabbit). Cut out the ears for the dog or pig only, and pin the two layers (one felt, one fabric) together for the cat or rabbit.

Mark and cut out the felt pieces for the faces and the base. With the very small pieces like the eye pupils it is easier sometimes to cut them free hand without marking first.

Machine or back stitch (*figs 4a, 4b, p 31*) around the dome of the body leaving the base open. Also stitch round the ears of the cat or rabbit. Cut out, leaving about $\frac{3}{8}$in (1cm) seam on the body and $\frac{1}{4}$in (5mm) on the ears. Clip the curves (*fig 11a*) and the points of the cat ears (*fig 11b*).

Turn the body through to the right side and stuff firmly. Run a gathering thread round the base of the body and pull up tight (*fig 12a*).

Stitch to hold (*fig 12b*). Pin the base pieces onto the body and hem stitch into position (*fig 13*).

Turn the cat or rabbit ears through to the right side. Turn the raw edges under and oversew together (*fig 14*). Place in position on the body and lay back. Stitch across the front then fold the ear forward over the stitching and stitch across the back (*figs 15a and 15b*). The ears for the dog and pig need only be stitched underneath as this makes the ear hang properly (*figs 16a and 16b*).

Embroider the noses and mouths onto the face pieces. Stitch the pupil onto the main eye piece and stitch three long stitches for eyelashes (*fig 17*). Pin the pieces onto the body using long pins to get the position right, then stitch into place (*fig 18*).

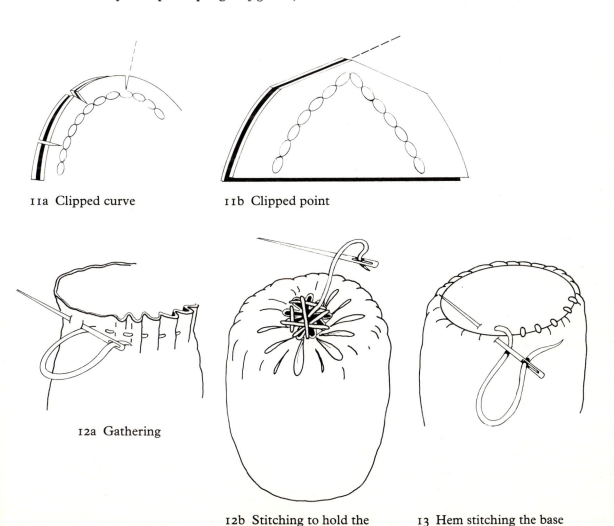

11a Clipped curve

11b Clipped point

12a Gathering

12b Stitching to hold the gathering

13 Hem stitching the base

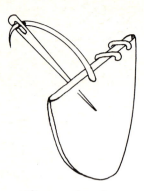

14 Oversewing the raw edges of the ears

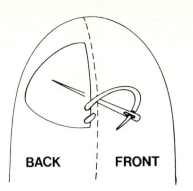

BACK   FRONT

15a Attaching the ears to the cat and rabbit

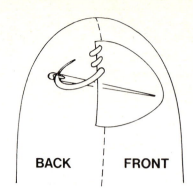

BACK   FRONT

15b

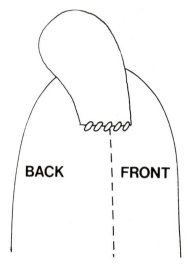

BACK   FRONT

16a Attaching the ears to the cat and rabbit

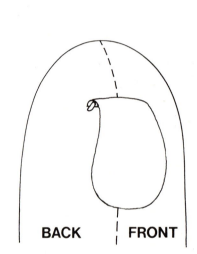

BACK   FRONT

16b

 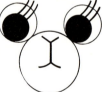 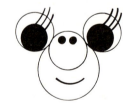

17 Faces: cat, rabbit, dog, pig

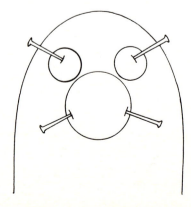

18 Pinning the eyes and face onto the body

36

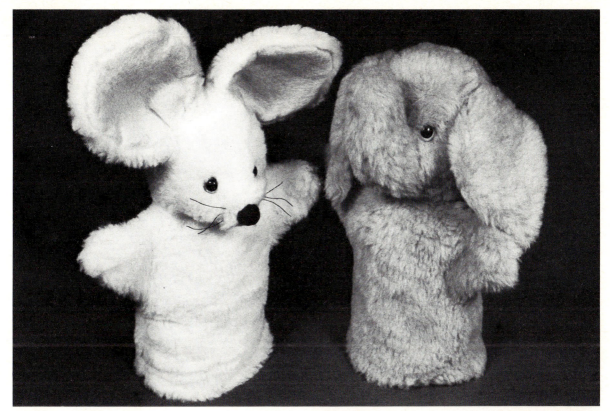

19 *Glove puppets: mouse, elephant, frog, penguin*

GLOVE PUPPETS
PENGUIN · FROG
ELEPHANT · MOUSE

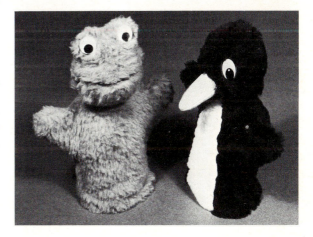

Puppets are for children of all ages (*19*) and once the basic idea is mastered it is possible to use heads from any similar sized animal pattern with the body pattern given here (Pattern 2).

Materials

Penguin
Black fur fabric, 10 in × 22 in (25 cm × 55cm)
White fur fabric, 8 in × 3 in (20 cm × 7 cm)
Yellow felt, 4 in × 3½ in (10 cm × 8 cm)
Oval eyes, ¾ in × 1¼ in (20 mm × 30 mm)

Frog
Green fur fabric, 10 in × 23 in (25 cm × 58 cm)
Moving eyes, ¾ in (20 mm)

Elephant
Grey fur fabric, 10 in × 23 in (25 cm × 78 cm)
Grey felt, 6 in × 8 in (15 cm × 20 cm)
Blue eyes, ⅝ in (16 mm)

Mouse
White fur fabric, 10 in × 30 in (25 cm × 75 cm)
Pink felt, 5 in × 9½ in (12 cm × 24 cm)
Blue eyes, ½ in (12 mm)
Scrap of black felt for nose
A few fine strands of unravelled nylon cord or fishing line for whiskers
Oddment of felt, 3¼ in × 5½ in (8 cm × 14 cm)
A few handfuls of stuffing
Matching thread

PATTERN 2

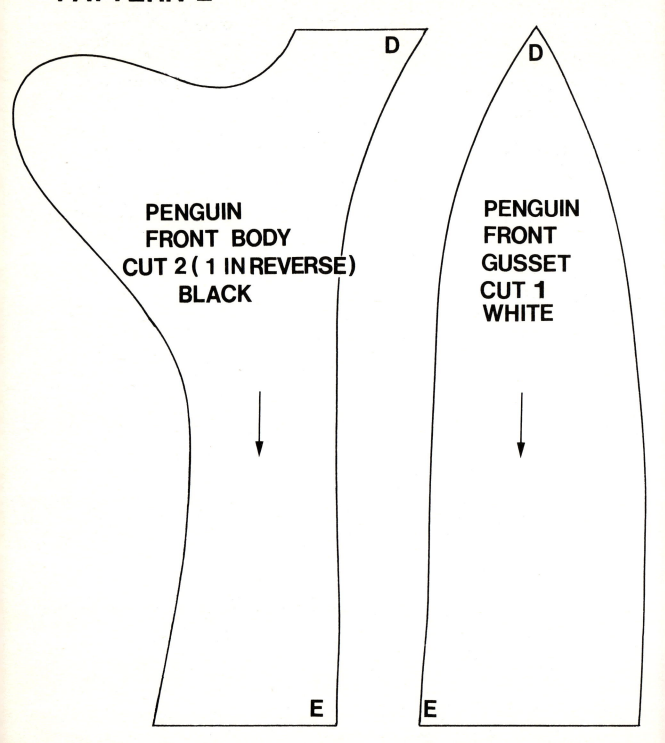

D

PENGUIN
FRONT BODY
CUT 2 (1 IN REVERSE)
BLACK

E

D

PENGUIN
FRONT
GUSSET
CUT 1
WHITE

E

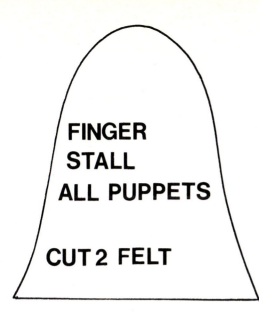

**FINGER
STALL
ALL PUPPETS**

CUT 2 FELT

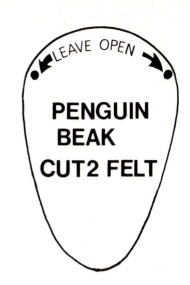

LEAVE OPEN

**PENGUIN
BEAK
CUT 2 FELT**

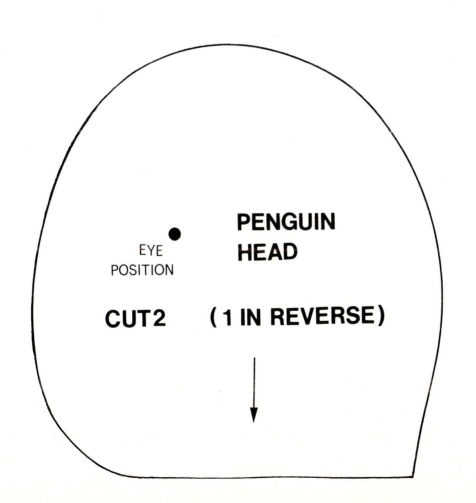

EYE
POSITION

**PENGUIN
HEAD**

CUT 2   (1 IN REVERSE)

PATTERN 2

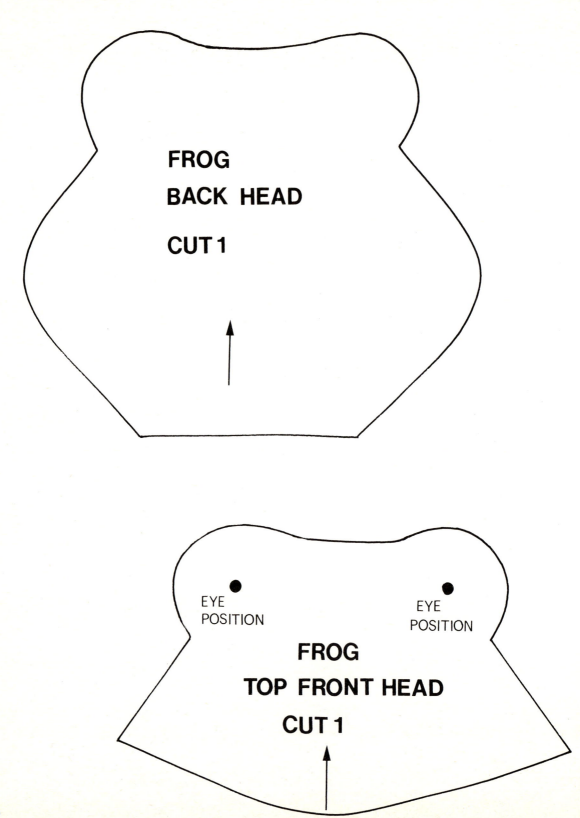

FROG
BACK HEAD
CUT 1

EYE
POSITION

EYE
POSITION

FROG
TOP FRONT HEAD
CUT 1

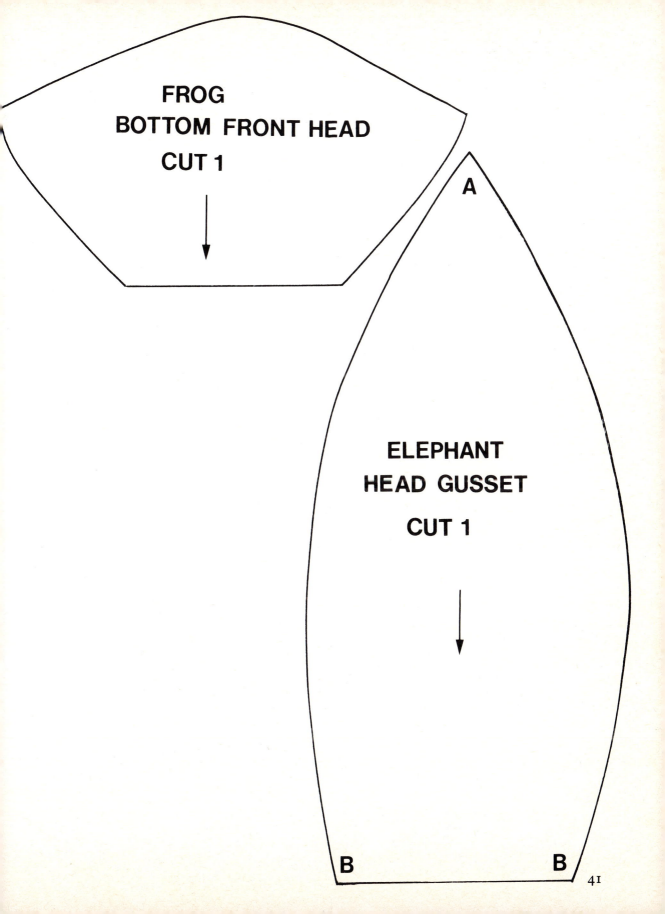

FROG
BOTTOM FRONT HEAD
CUT 1

A

ELEPHANT
HEAD GUSSET

CUT 1

B   B

41

PATTERN 2

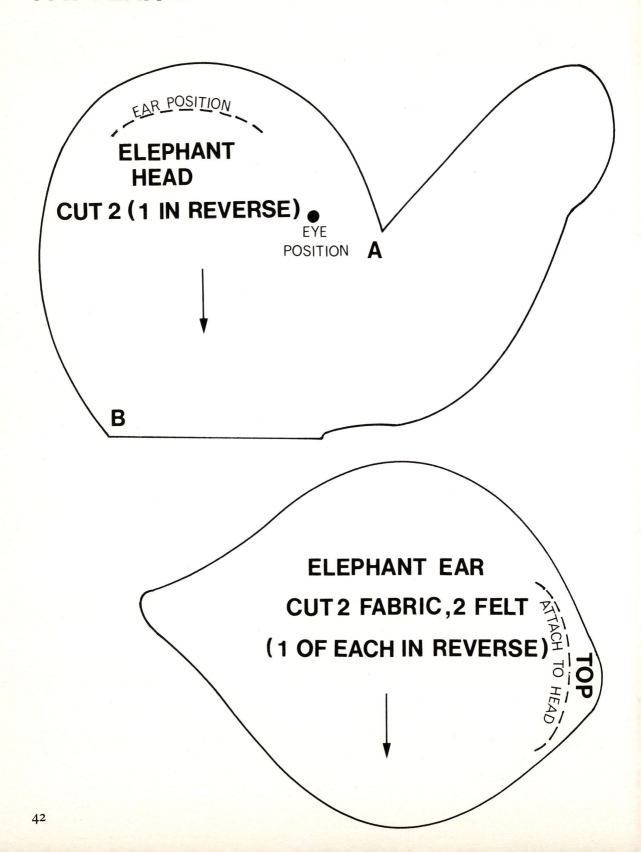

EAR POSITION

ELEPHANT HEAD

CUT 2 (1 IN REVERSE)

EYE POSITION

A

B

ELEPHANT EAR

CUT 2 FABRIC, 2 FELT

(1 OF EACH IN REVERSE)

ATTACH TO HEAD

TOP

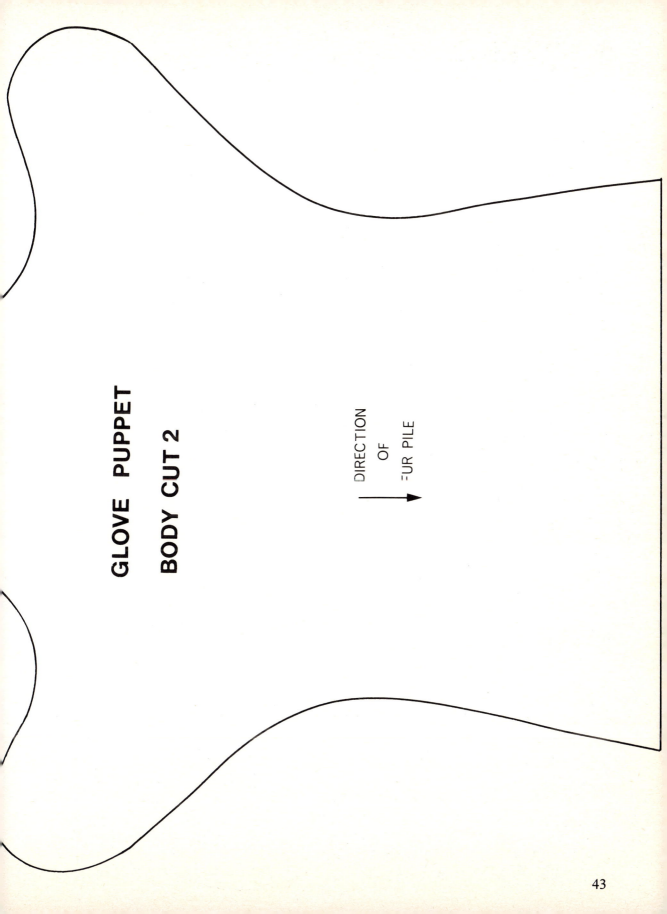

GLOVE PUPPET

BODY CUT 2

DIRECTION

OF

FUR PILE

→

PATTERN 2

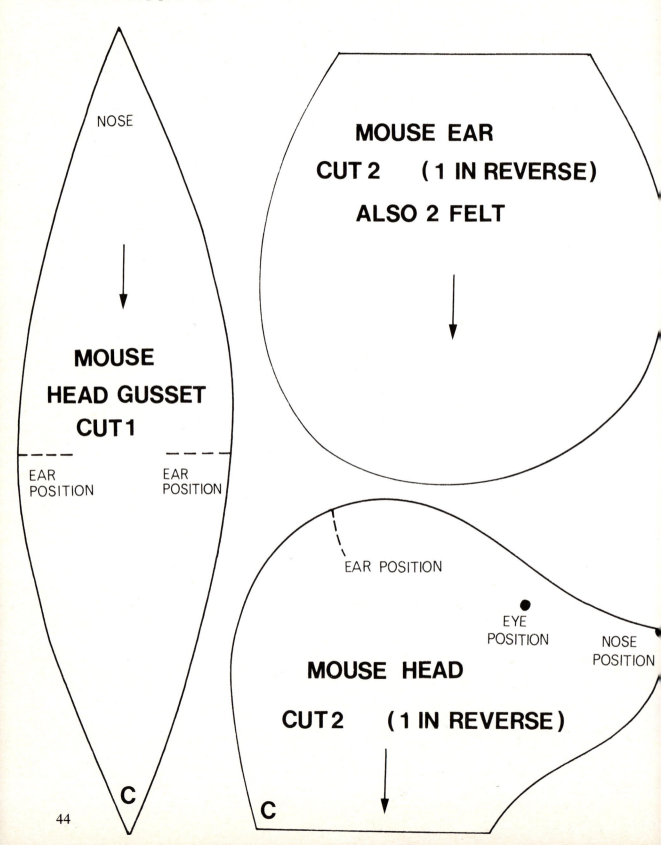

NOSE

MOUSE EAR

CUT 2   (1 IN REVERSE)

ALSO 2 FELT

MOUSE

HEAD GUSSET

CUT 1

EAR
POSITION

EAR
POSITION

EAR POSITION

EYE
POSITION

NOSE
POSITION

MOUSE HEAD

CUT 2   (1 IN REVERSE)

C

C

44

Instructions

Check the direction of the pile of the fur and lay out the pattern pieces accordingly. Draw round the pieces, marking one piece in reverse where indicated. Cut out carefully along the drawn lines parting the fur as you go. Also mark and cut out the felt pieces.

Pin, oversew and back stitch (or machine) the two body pieces together leaving the neck and the base open. The front body of the penguin is in three pieces, to be joined first. Turn up about $\frac{1}{4}$in (5mm) around the bottom and hem to the inside (fig 7, p 31).

Pin, oversew and back stitch (or machine) the head pieces. The mouse and elephant have two side head pieces and a head gusset. The frog has a back head and two front head pieces. The penguin has two side head pieces (fig 20).

Attach the eyes (see p 31).

Turn the head through to the right side and stuff firmly, but leaving sufficient room in the head to place two fingers. Cut two pieces for the finger stall in felt and back stitch or machine round the edge leaving the base open (fig 21).

Place this in the head and oversew round the neck (fig 22). Place the head inside the body with the nose facing the front, and pin, oversew and back stitch round the neck (fig 23). In order to do this the head will have to be considerably squashed, but can be pulled into shape again afterwards. Although this is the neatest and strongest way to finish the neck, it is not possible to attach the head of the elephant in the same way because the trunk gets in the way. For the elephant, turn the body also to the right side and stitching the head and body alternately, work round the neck several times

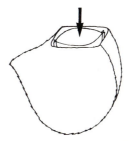

22 Placing the finger stall in the head

20 Construction of head
a Mouse b Elephant c Frog
d Penguin

GUSSET

21 Finger stall

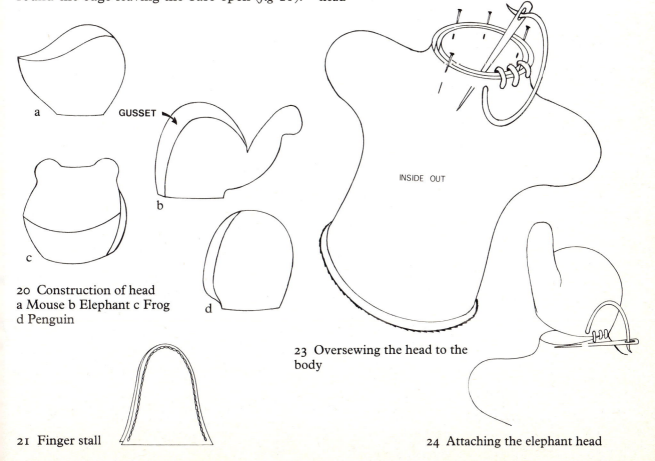

INSIDE OUT

23 Oversewing the head to the body

24 Attaching the elephant head

45

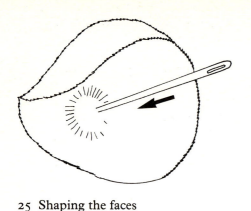

25 Shaping the faces

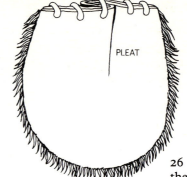

26 Oversewing the raw edges of the mouse ears

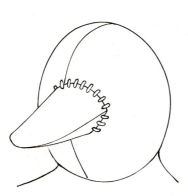

27 Attaching the penguin beak

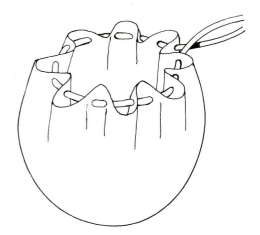

28 Gathering the mouse nose

(*fig 24*). Reshape all the faces using a toy maker's needle or long darner (*fig 25*).

For the elephant and mouse, trim the felt ear pieces slightly smaller than the fur pieces then pin, oversew and back stitch or machine the two pieces together. Turn the elephant ears through and ladder stitch the opening (*fig 5, p 31*). Turn the mouse ears through then pleat and oversew the edges (*fig 26*). Position the ears on the head and lay back; stitch the felt side first. Fold the ears over the stitching and stitch the fur side as well (*figs 15a and 15b, p 36*).

Back stitch or machine the two beak pieces together for the penguin leaving it open at the wide end. Turn through and stuff. Stitch round the open end directly onto the head (*fig 27*). For the mouse nose cut a circle of black felt approximately 1¼in (3cm) in diameter. Run a gathering thread round the edge and draw up slightly (*fig 28*). Stuff the nose and draw up the thread tightly and stitch to hold. Stitch into position on the face.

Using a toy maker's needle or long darner and with two strands of black double knitting wool, embroider the mouth on the mouse and frog. To make whiskers for the mouse, tie a knot about 2in (5cm) from one end of a piece of fine nylon. Using a long needle thread the whisker through the face so that 1¼in (3cm) remain on one side. Tie a knot the other side and trim to 1¼in (3cm). Make two more whiskers the same.

TEDDY OR PANDA

The teddy bear has become such a traditional favourite that it is impossible to have a collection of toys without including one (29). With a few simple variations this bear pattern is also used to make a panda (Pattern 3).

Materials

Panda Black fur fabric, 10in × 16in (25cm × 40cm)
White fur fabric, 10in × 16in (25cm × 40cm)
Black felt, 3in × 6in (7cm × 15cm)

Teddy Fur fabric, 10 in × 32in (25cm × 80cm)
Matching felt, 3in × 4in (7cm × 10cm)
Approx. 1lb (or 500g) stuffing
Eyes, ½in (12mm)
Scrap of felt for nose
2 strands of double knitting wool for mouth

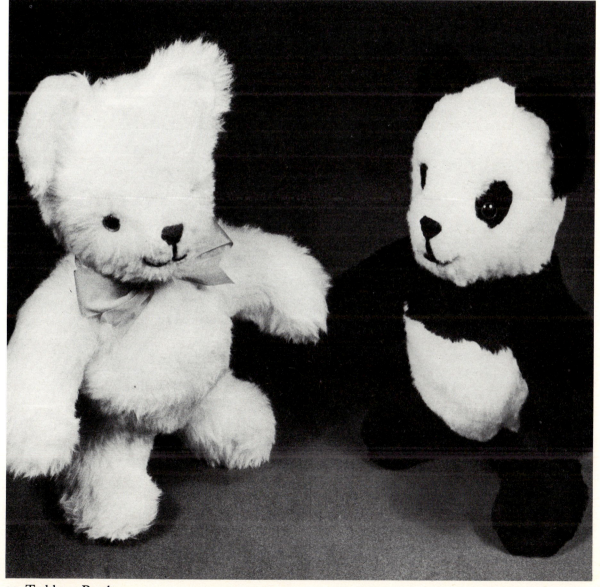

29 Teddy or Panda

PATTERN 3

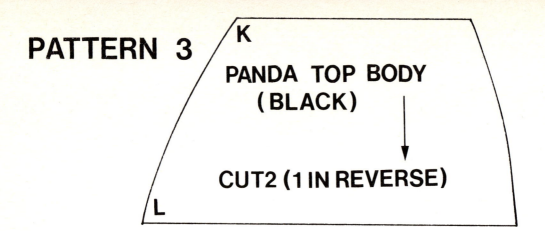

K

**PANDA TOP BODY
(BLACK)**

CUT 2 (1 IN REVERSE)

L

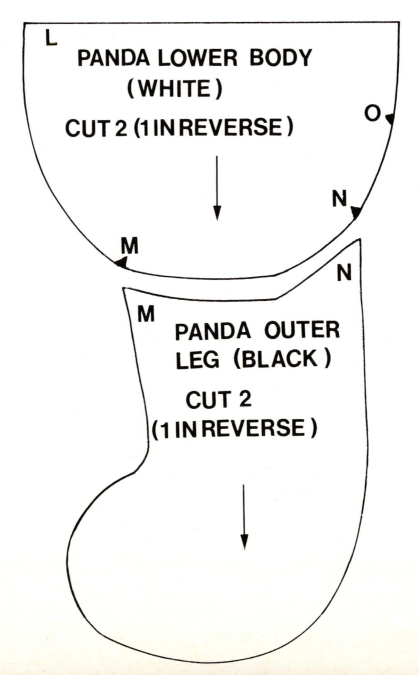

L

**PANDA LOWER BODY
(WHITE)**

CUT 2 (1 IN REVERSE)

O

N

M

N

M

**PANDA OUTER
LEG (BLACK)**

**CUT 2
(1 IN REVERSE)**

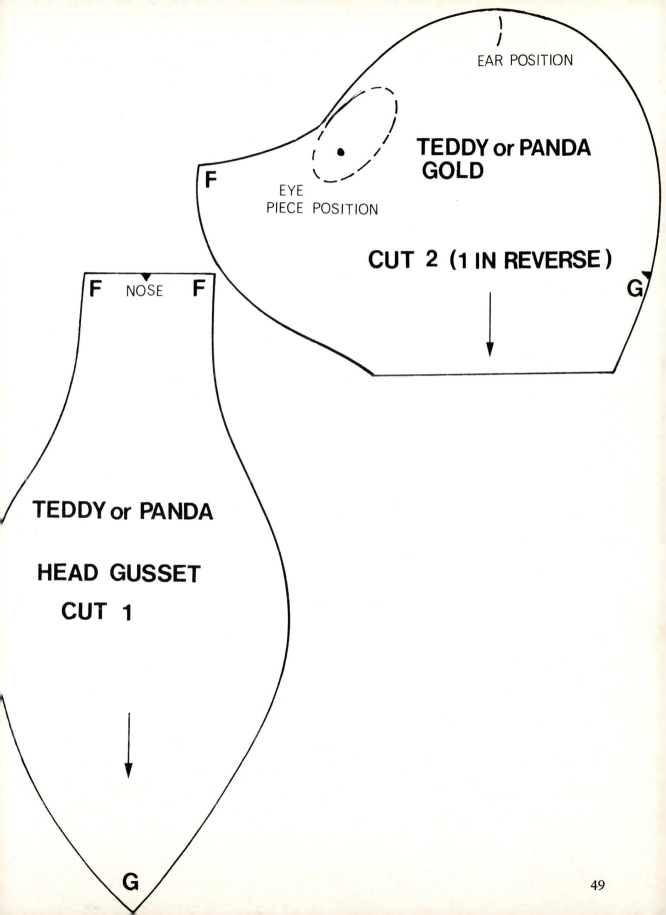

EAR POSITION

TEDDY or PANDA
GOLD

F

EYE
PIECE POSITION

CUT 2 (1 IN REVERSE)

G

F   NOSE   F

TEDDY or PANDA

HEAD GUSSET

CUT 1

G

49

PATTERN 3

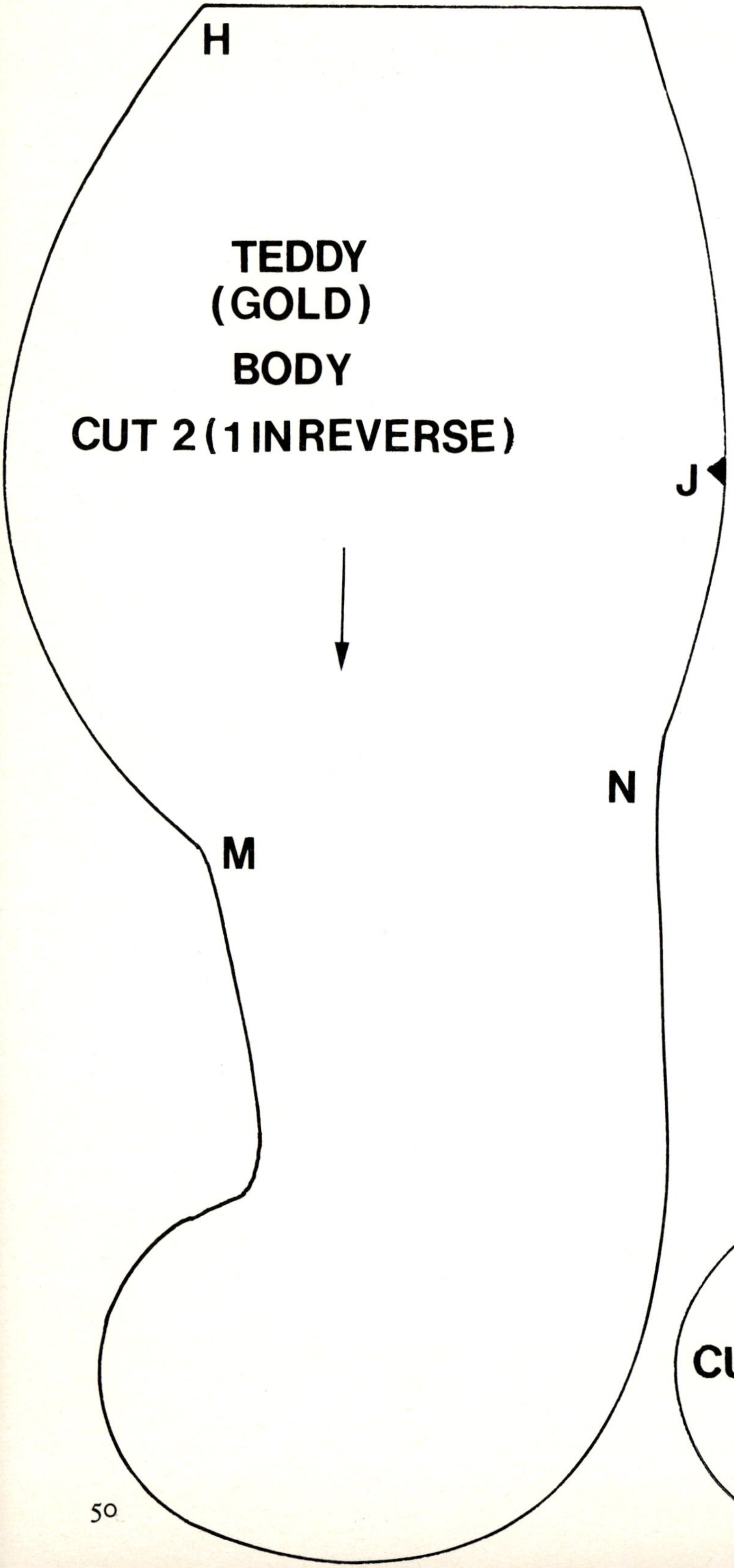

H

**TEDDY
(GOLD)
BODY
CUT 2 (1 IN REVERSE)**

J

N

M

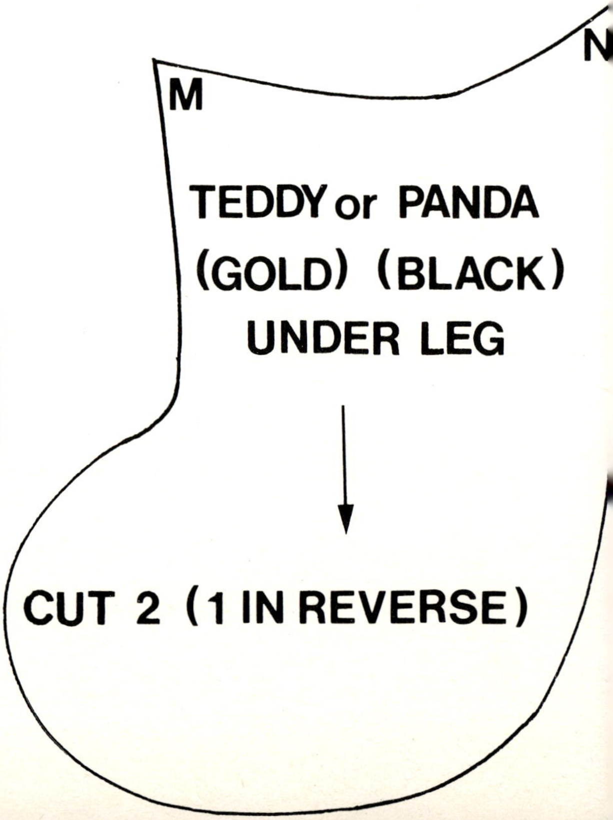

M

N

**TEDDY or PANDA
(GOLD) (BLACK)
UNDER LEG**

CUT 2 (1 IN REVERSE)

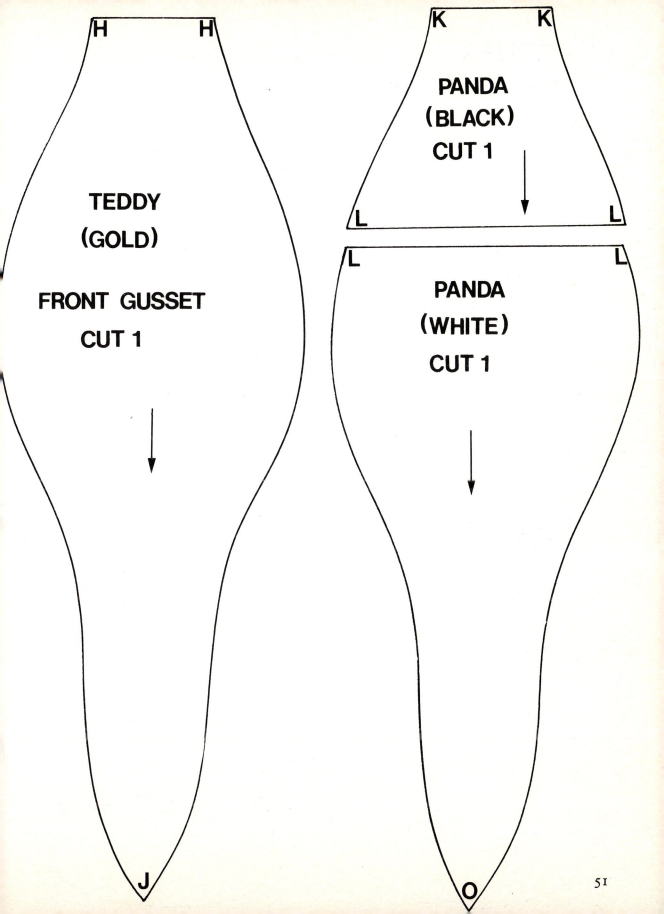

H   H

TEDDY

(GOLD)

FRONT GUSSET

CUT 1

J

K   K

PANDA

(BLACK)

CUT 1

L   L

L   L

PANDA

(WHITE)

CUT 1

O

PATTERN 3

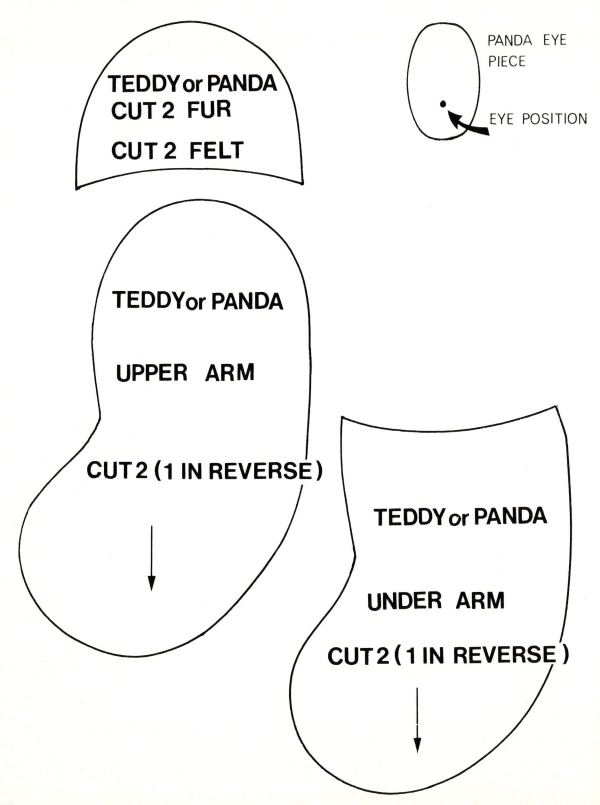

TEDDY or PANDA
CUT 2 FUR

CUT 2 FELT

PANDA EYE
PIECE

EYE POSITION

TEDDY or PANDA

UPPER ARM

CUT 2 (1 IN REVERSE)

TEDDY or PANDA

UNDER ARM

CUT 2 (1 IN REVERSE)

52

Instructions

Head

Check the direction of the pile of the fur and lay out the pattern pieces accordingly. Draw round the pieces, marking one piece in reverse where indicated. Cut out carefully along the drawn lines parting the fur as you go. Also mark and cut out the felt pieces. Pin, oversew and back stitch (or machine) the gusset into the head (fig 30), and the back of the head below the gusset. Pin, oversew and back stitch (or machine) from the nose to the neck at the front, folding the nose of the gusset in half (fig 31).

Eyes

TEDDY Attach safety eyes in position marked then turn through to right side.

PANDA Attach safety eyes through both felt pieces and head (fig 32); turn through and stitch the felt onto the head. Stuff the head firmly. Run a gathering thread round the neck and draw up; fasten off (figs 12a and 12b, p 35). Stitch on the nose and with a toy maker's needle or long darner embroider the mouth (fig 33).

Ears

Trim the felt pieces slightly smaller than the fur pieces. Pin and sew the pieces together leaving the bottom open. Turn through and oversew along the edges pulling up slightly so that the ear curves (figs 34a and 34b). Position the ears on the head and lay back; stitch the felt side first. Fold the ears forward over the stitching and stitch the fur side as well (figs 15a and 15b, p 36).

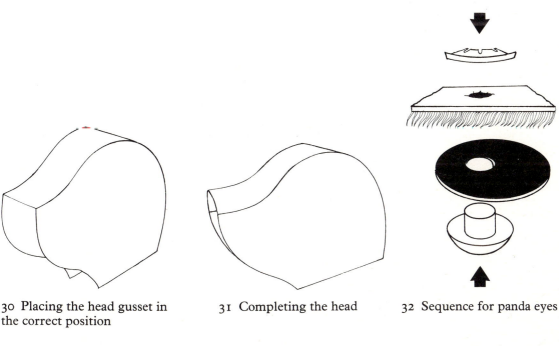

30 Placing the head gusset in the correct position

31 Completing the head

32 Sequence for panda eyes

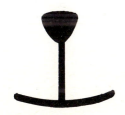

33 Nose and mouth for panda and teddy

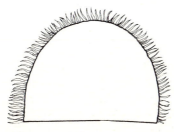

34a Oversewing the raw edges of the ears

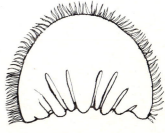

34b Oversewing the raw edges of the ears

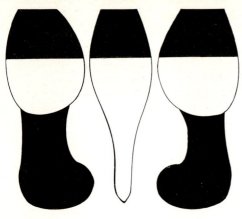

35 Making up the body pieces
for the panda

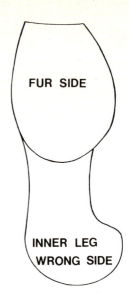

FUR SIDE

INNER LEG
WRONG SIDE

36 Attaching the inner leg

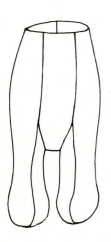

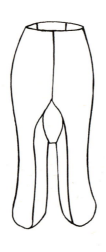

FRONT   BACK

37 Position of body gusset

Body

PANDA First pin and sew the gusset pieces together and then the body and leg pieces (*fig 35*). Pin and sew the inner leg pieces to the body pieces (*fig 36*). Pin and sew the gusset in position (*fig 37*). Continue to pin and sew up the back so that only the neck is left open. Turn through and stuff the body firmly, paying particular attention to the feet and the point where the legs join the body. Run a gathering thread round the neck and draw up. Fasten off. Attach the head to the body by holding firmly and stitching alternately into the head and body with strong thread. Work round the neck two

or three times in this way until the head is quite firm (*fig 24, p 45*).

Arms

Pin and sew the arm pieces together leaving them open at the top. Turn through and stuff firmly. Attach to the body in the same way as the head (*fig 24, p 45*).

Finishing off

Pick out any fur caught in the seams using a long pin. Being careful not to overdo it, trim the fur around the nose and mouth. Brush the whole animal with a wire brush.

RAG DOLLS

These two simple basic dolls (Pattern 4) can be varied in many ways. They can be given different faces or colouring. Short fluffy hair can be made by using fur fabric and the hair base pattern. The trousers and dress could be made ankle length. All kinds of trimmings and ribbons could be used to give quite a different effect (38).

Materials

(quantities are given for each item so that oddments can be used)
Calico, 8in × 32in
(20cm × 80cm) for
each doll

Wool for hair
Felt to match hair,
7in × 3in (18cm × 7cm
Thread for sewing and for features
Stuffing
Small lengths of elastic
Dress: cotton fabric, 13in × 9½in (32cm × 24cm)
Knickers: cotton fabric, 6¼in × 6in (16cm × 15cm)
Shirt: cotton fabric, 13in × 5in (32cm × 13cm)

Trousers: felt, 6in × 6½in (16cm × 15cm)
Shoes: felt 3in × 3½in (7cm × 8cm)
Boots: felt 3in × 5in (7cm × 12cm)

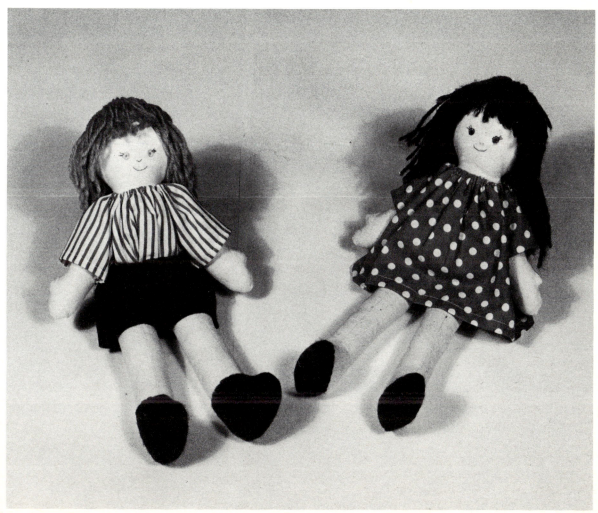

38 Rag dolls

PATTERN 4

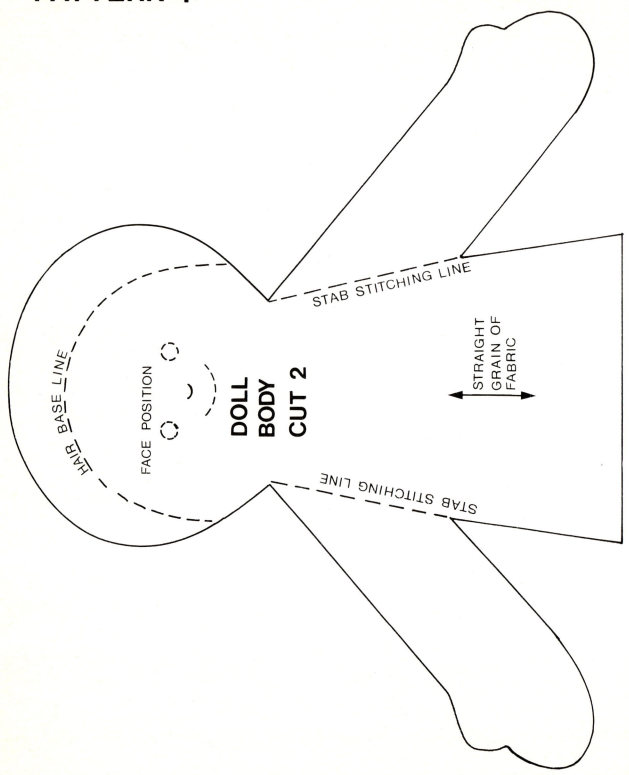

STAB STITCHING LINE

HAIR BASE LINE

FACE POSITION

DOLL
BODY
CUT 2

STRAIGHT GRAIN OF FABRIC

STAB STITCHING LINE

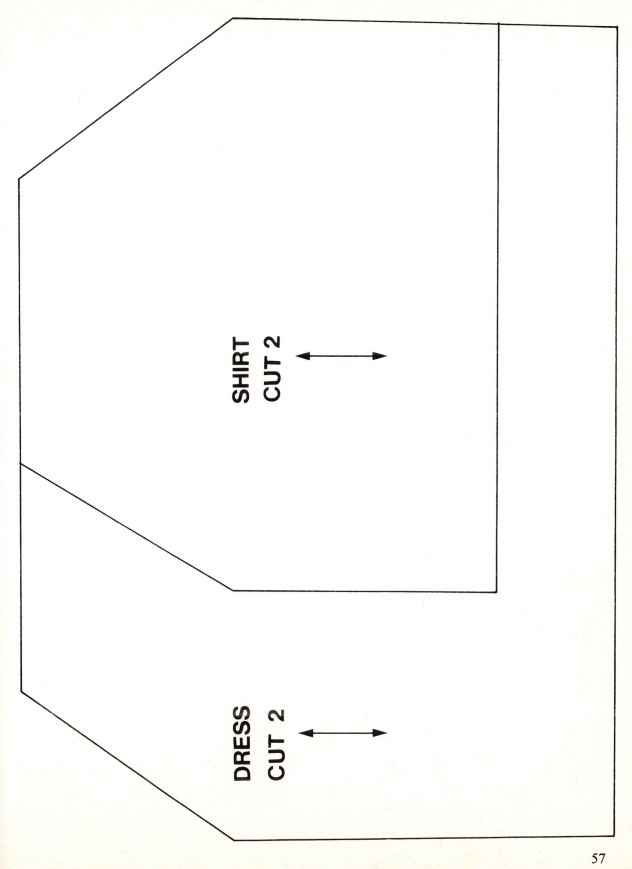

SHIRT
CUT 2

DRESS
CUT 2

PATTERN 4

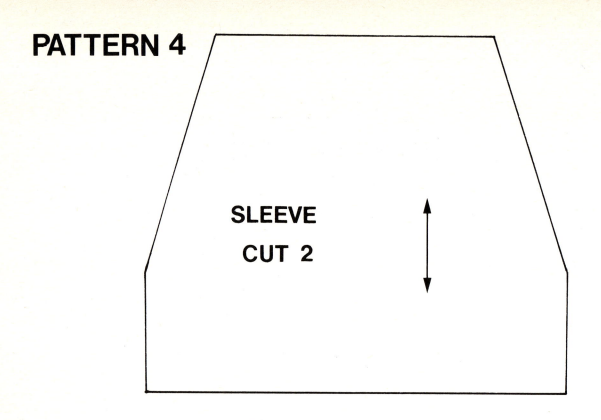

SLEEVE

CUT 2

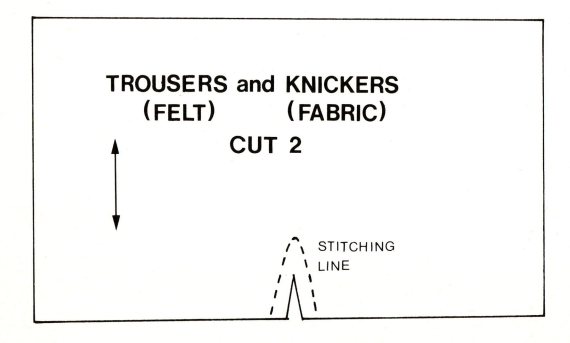

TROUSERS and KNICKERS
(FELT)   (FABRIC)

CUT 2

STITCHING
LINE

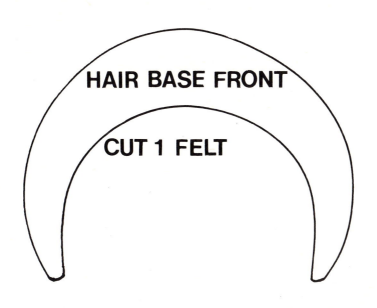

HAIR BASE FRONT

CUT 1 FELT

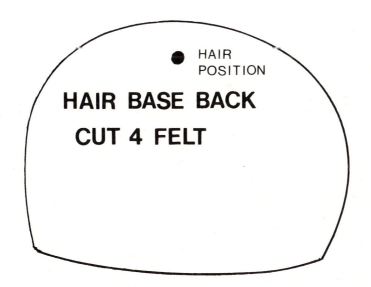

HAIR
POSITION

HAIR BASE BACK

CUT 4 FELT

PATTERN 4

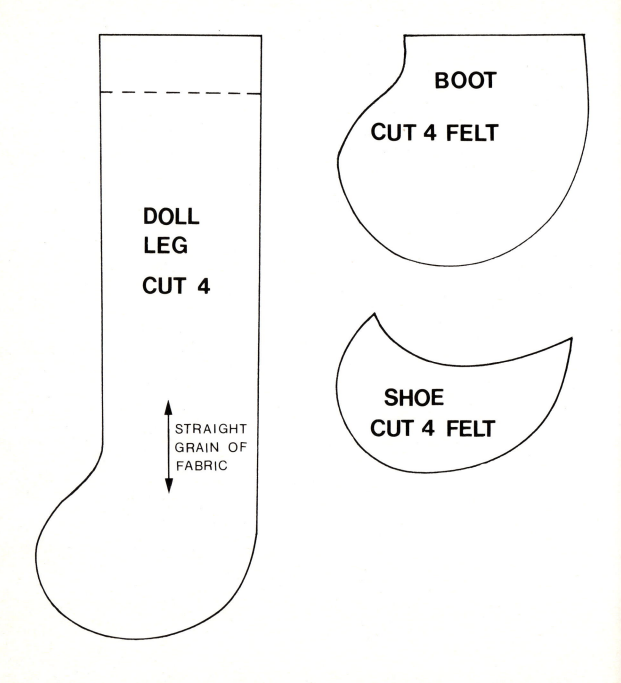

DOLL
LEG

CUT 4

STRAIGHT
GRAIN OF
FABRIC

BOOT

CUT 4 FELT

SHOE
CUT 4 FELT

Instructions

Bodies

Fold the calico in half so that it measures 8in × 16in (20cm × 40cm). Lay on the two pattern pieces, following the grain of the fabric and draw round the patterns with a pencil. Repeat the leg pattern once more. The drawn line is the stitching line so do not cut out. Pin round inside the drawn lines to hold the two layers together. Machine or back stitch round the drawn lines leaving them open at the bottom of the body and at the top of the legs.

Cut round, leaving approximately $\frac{1}{2}$in (10mm) seams. Clip round the curves of the feet, hands, head and into the points at neck, arm and thumb (*fig 39*). Turn through.

Stuff the arms firmly to the point where they join the body. Stab stitch or machine using a zip foot across the top of the arm in the position shown on the pattern (*fig 6, p 31*). This allows the arms to move when the body is stuffed.

Stuff the legs to within $\frac{1}{2}$in (10mm) of the top. Stab stitch across to hold the stuffing in (*fig 40*). Back stitch the legs onto the front body (*fig 41*). Stuff the head and body. Fold the legs down and turn to the back. Turn the back body piece under and hem across (*fig 42*).

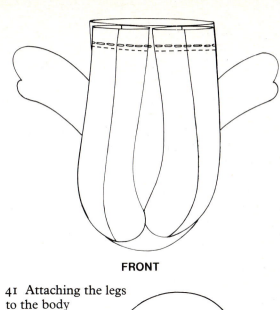

FRONT

41 Attaching the legs to the body

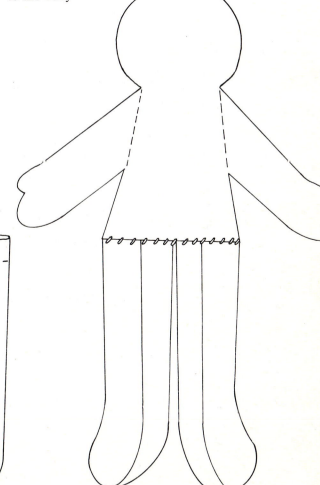

BACK

42 Hemming across the back of the body after stuffing

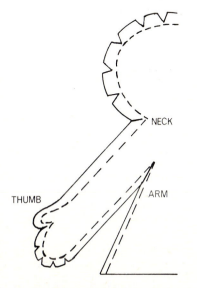

NECK

THUMB

ARM

39 Clipping the curves and points

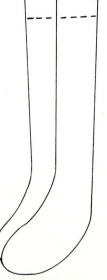

40 Stab stitching on the leg

Faces
Using the diagram (*fig 43*) as a guide, embroider the faces in coloured sewing cotton.

Hair
Mark and cut out the two felt pieces for the hair base. Back stitch or machine the two pieces together and hem into position on the head (*fig 44*).

Cut 100 strands of wool 8in (20cm) long (for boy) and 10in (25cm) long (for girl). Bind tightly in the middle with a piece of the same wool (*fig 45*). Fan out half the strands onto the head with the bound part on the position given (*fig 46*). Stitch this centre securely to the head and catch the fanned-out strands here and there. Fan out the remaining half of the woollen strands and catch them into position every so often following the edge of the felt hair base. Trim the fringe and then the rest of the hair evenly round.

Mark and cut out the pieces for the clothes.

Dress and shirt
With right sides together, pin and back stitch or machine the sleeves to the body pieces taking a $\frac{1}{8}$in (3mm) seam (*fig 47*). Still with the right sides together pin and back stitch or machine the sleeve and side seams with $\frac{1}{8}$in (3mm) seams

(*fig 48*). Turn a $\frac{1}{4}$in (6mm) hem round the neck, pin and either hem or machine leaving a small gap for the elastic. Using a large round-ended needle or bodkin, thread the elastic through the neck hem, pull up to the neck size and knot the two ends together. Hem or machine along the gap. Turn a $\frac{3}{8}$in (8mm) hem at the bottom, pin and hem stitch or machine. Turn a $\frac{3}{8}$in (8mm) hem at the bottom of each sleeve. Pin and hem stitch round (the sleeve is too small for the machine).

Knickers and trousers
Pin, back stitch or machine the side seams and the centre V. Clip the V. Turn a $\frac{1}{4}$in (6mm) hem round the waist, pin, hem stitch or machine leaving a gap for the elastic. Insert the elastic as for the neck and then hem stitch or machine the gap.

For the knickers only, turn $\frac{1}{4}$in (6mm) hems round both legs, pin and hem stitch leaving gaps for elastic. Insert the elastic in each leg as before.

Boots and shoes
Pin and back stitch or machine round the two pieces for each foot leaving the top open. Turn through, place on the foot and hem stitch into position.

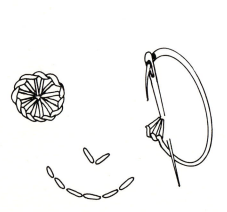

43 Faces

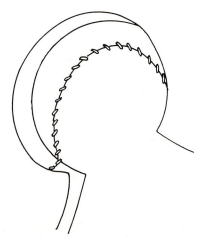

44 Attaching the hair base

45 Binding the hair strands

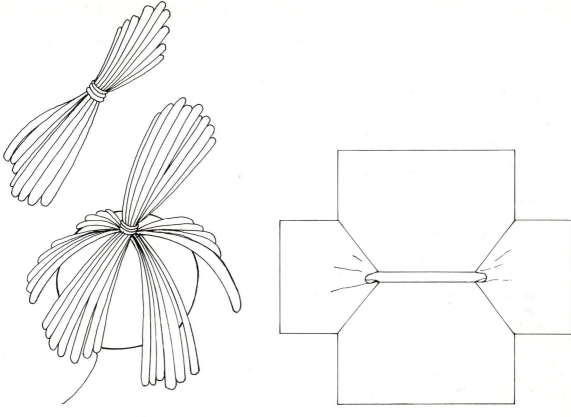

46 Positioning the hair

47 Making up the dress and shirt

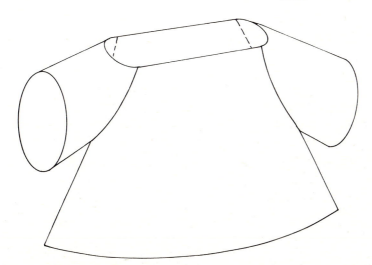

48 Dress and shirt with side seams stitched

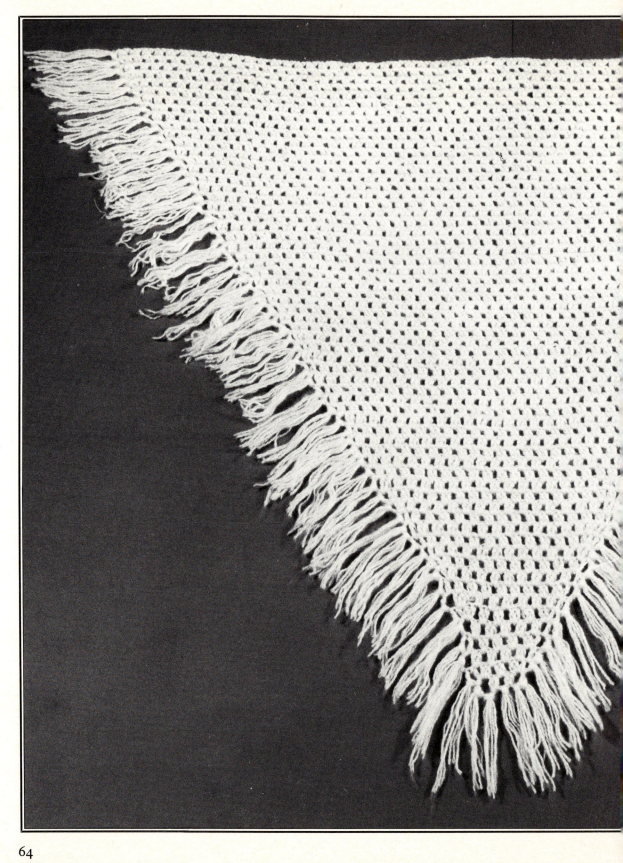

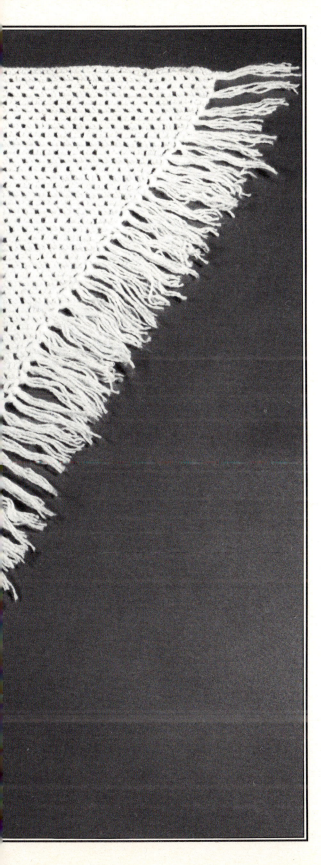

3 Knitting and Crochet

These two traditionally related crafts may not at first appear to be suitable for disabled people as one tends to assume that two able hands are called for. With the use of a vice they can easily be adapted for someone who only has the use of one hand. A person who has previous knowledge of either knitting or crochet prior to the occurrence of their disability will of course find these crafts easier than someone who has not, but this should not prevent the latter from becoming equally competent. Many people watch television or read a book and knit at the same time thus indicating that poor sight is not too much of a handicap. Plenty of blind people are superb knitters.

The instructions given here will be for the basic stitches using a vice clamped to a table. We have only included a few patterns, as once the technique is mastered ordinary commercial patterns can be followed. Large print patterns are available for those with poor eye-sight (see p 116)

You may notice in this chapter that there are more patterns given for crochet than for knitting; this is because generally knitting patterns are more widely available, although crochet is becoming more popular.

EQUIPMENT

A selection of *steel knitting needles*, the longer the better if used in a vice. Plastic ones are too unstable.

A selection of *steel crochet hooks*. If using a vice a Tunisian hook is longer and gives more room to manoeuvre.

A vice is useful to clamp the needle in position when working with one hand.

Elastic bands are useful to steady the knitting needle.

A Shetland knitting pad can also be used to steady the needles (see p 116 and *fig 1*).

A large tapestry needle for stitching up.

A bowl or box to keep the yarn in, to stop it rolling off the table.

A cork or *pin cushion* to hold the needle still while threading.

Scissors People with arthritic or weak hands will find Stirex scissors very useful. They require very little pressure to work and are much less tiring on the hands.

MATERIALS

There is a good range of yarns available at any wool shop. Nylon strips known as Nytrim are useful and can be bought cheaply from most handicraft suppliers.

NOTES ON TENSION FOR KNITTING AND CROCHET

It is always best to try out a small square of the pattern that you are going to use to see if your tension corresponds with the one given at the beginning of the instructions. It is particularly necessary when using a vice to hold the hook or needle.

If your sample square is too small compared with the given tension then try another one using a larger hook or needle. If it is too large then use a smaller hook or needle. It is worth the extra time before starting a garment to ensure good results.

You can also make your patterns larger or smaller by adding more stitches relevant to the tension. With square shaped garments, like the children's jumpers, this should not be too difficult to calculate.

KNITTING

Aids
If there is some feeling in both hands but not very much strength, knitting can be simply carried out by securing the needles to the wrists by elastic bands. This ensures that the needles cannot be dropped.

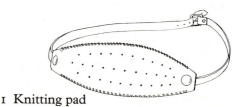

1 Knitting pad

There is also a knitting pad (*fig 1*) which comes from the Shetland Isles, where the knitters use it for complicated patterns. The end of one of the needles is placed into one of the holes; this steadies it and would enable someone with little feeling on one side to knit using the other hand, although the supported needle still needs to be held while knitting.

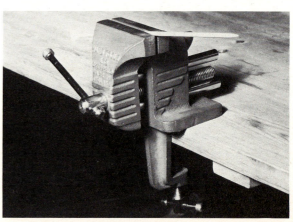

2 Vice holding knitting needle

Using a vice

The instructions here are for someone who is right handed; they should be reversed for a person using their left hand.

Place one of the needles in the vice pointing to the right at a slight angle (*fig 2*).

Casting on

The easiest way to cast on is by using the needle in the vice and your hand. Make a slip loop and place on needle then take the wool from the front and over the needle (*fig 3a*). Take the loop now made with the thumb and index finger and slide it to the end of the needle. Slip it off and turn it once placing it back on the needle, on stitch formed. Repeat until number of stitches required are on needle (*fig 3b*).

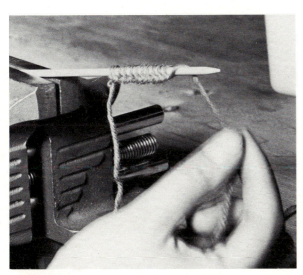

3a Casting on

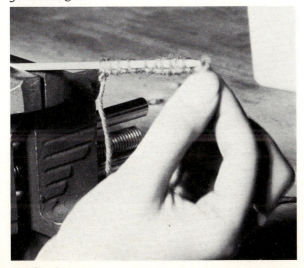

3b Casting on

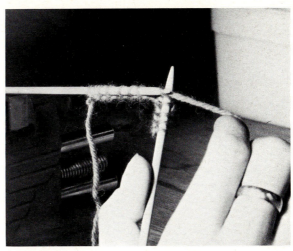

4a Knitting a row

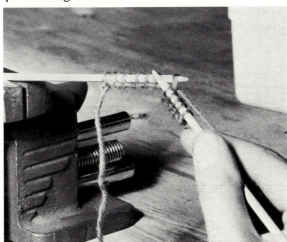

4b Knitting a row

To knit a row

Place the point of the needle in your hand into the first stitch on the needle in the vice. Holding the wool in the right hand wrap it round the point of the needle in your hand, draw the wool through the first stitch on the vice needle then slip this stitch off. Repeat this with each stitch until the row is knitted (*figs 4a and 4b*). For the first stitch you may find that you have to just support the end of the needle you are holding with your chest or shoulder while you wrap the wool round. This is not necessary with the other stitches as both needles become attached to the work and this supports them.

At the end of the row all the stitches will be on the needle in your hand, so you have to swop the needles over, putting the full one in the vice.

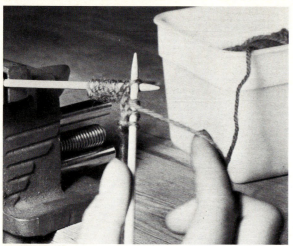

5a Purling a row

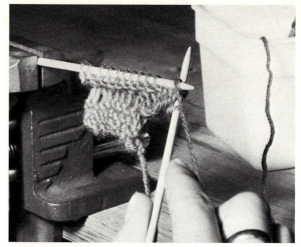

6a Spider stitch

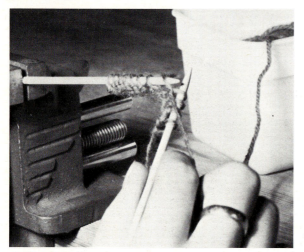

5b Purling a row

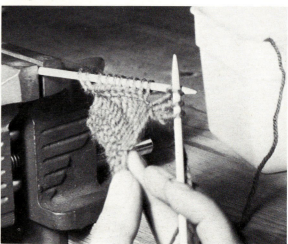

6b Spider stitch

To purl a row

Place the needle in your hand into the front of the first stitch (*figs 5a and 5b*). Take the wool from the front of the work and wrap it over and round the point of the needle just inserted. Draw the wool through with the needle to the back of the work, then slip the stitch off the vice needle. Repeat to the end of row.

Increasing

To increase, knit a stitch as normal but do not slip it off the needle; then knit into the back loop, so that you then have two stitches.

Decreasing

To decrease, slip one stitch onto the needle in hand, knit the next stitch. Then pass the slip stitch back over the knitted one.

Spider stitch

Place the needle in as for a knit row. Wind the wool round both points of the needles and then knit one (*figs 6a and 6b*).

KNITTED SHOPPING BAG

Materials
Nytrim, 12oz (350gm) ball
Large pair of wooden needles, no. 00
No 2.50 crochet hook

Bag
Cast on 25 stitches. Knit 1 row plain. Knit 34 rows in spider stitch. Knit 1 row plain. Cast off.

Handles
(See p 72 for an explanation of crochet terms.)
Join on yarn at one end of cast-on edge.
With crochet hook work 25 ch.
ss to other end of same edge work, 2 dc into end.
Turn work, 1 ch 24 dc over 25 chain already formed, with the last dc into original starting point.
Repeat on other edge.
On wrong side ladder stitch sides of bag, leaving 6 rows of knitting free at the top of bag.
Sew in all loose ends.

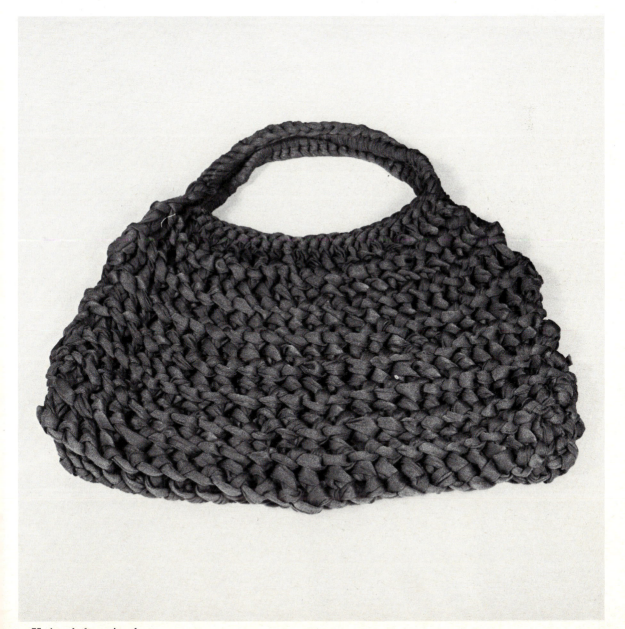

7 Knitted shopping bag

CHILD'S MULTI-COLOURED JUMPER

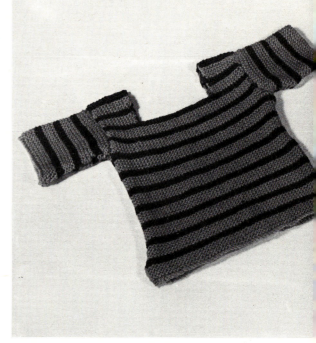

Size

Body length 12, 14, 16in (31, 35, 39cm)
Chest 18, 20, 22in (46, 51, 54cm)

Materials

Hermit Double Knitting 100% wool, 1oz (or 25g) balls:
(3, 4, 4) Kingfisher (KF)
(1, 2, 2) White (W)
1 ball each of Copper (C), Tan (T), Amber (A), Gold (G)
2 small buttons to match KF
No 9 knitting needles

Tension

10 st and 16 rows to 2in (5cm)

Body

Make 2 the same, as follows:
Cast on (51, 56, 61) stitches, using KF
Knit (22, 36, 50) rows
Knit (2 rows C, 2 rows KF) 3 times
Knit (2 rows T, 2 rows KF) 3 times
Knit (2 rows A, 2 rows KF) twice
Knit (2 rows G, 2 rows KF) twice
Knit (2 rows W, 2 rows KF) twice
Knit 4 rows C
Knit 4 rows T
Knit 4 rows A
Knit 4 rows G
Knit 8 rows W
Knit 2 rows KF
Knit 2 rows W
Knit 2 rows KF
Knit 12 rows W
Knit 4 rows KF
Working on the first (11, 12, 13) stitches only, knit 7 rows KF then cast off.
Cast off centre stitches (29, 32, 35). Working on stitches left on needle (11, 12, 13), knit 7 rows KF then cast off.

Sleeve

Make 2 the same, as follows:
Using KF, cast on (32, 38, 44) stitches.
Knit (6, 10, 14) rows
Knit 2 rows C
Knit 2 rows KF

Knit 2 rows T
Knit 2 rows KF
Knit 2 rows A
Knit 2 rows KF
Knit 2 rows G
Knit 2 rows KF
Knit 2 rows W
Knit 2 rows KF
Knit 2 rows C
Knit 2 rows T
Knit 2 rows A
Knit 2 rows G
Knit 8 rows W
Cast off.
Sew in ends on wrong side.
Using oversewing with right sides facing, stitch up one shoulder completely, then sew only ¾in (2cm) of the other one (this will be a buttoned opening).
Lay flat and stitch sleeves on; try to match the white.
Stitch up arm and side seams, leaving ¾in (2cm) open at the bottom edge of the side seams.

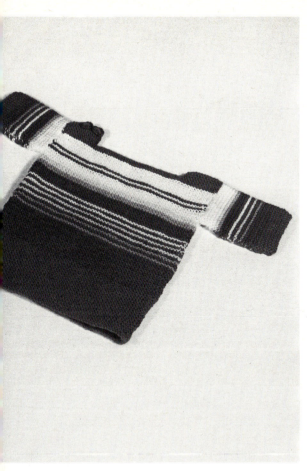

Make 2 button loops on the unstitched shoulder seam.
Sew on buttons. Damp press.

CHILD'S TWO-COLOUR STRIPED JUMPER

Size
Body length 12, 14, 16in (31, 35, 39cm)
Chest 18, 20, 22in (46, 51, 54cm)

Materials
Hermit Double Knitting 100% wool:
(4, 4, 5) 1oz (or 25g) balls Mustard (M)
2 × 1oz (or 25g) balls Emerald Green (G)
No 9 knitting needles

Tension
10 stitches and 16 rows to 2in (5cm)

Body
Make 2 the same, as follows:

Cast on (51, 56, 61) stitches.
Knit 8 rows M
Knit 4 rows G
Repeat these 12 rows until (6, 7, 8) green stripes are knitted.

Sleeve
Make 2 the same, as follows:
Using M, cast on (32, 38, 44) stitches.
Knit (8 rows M, 4 rows G) 3 times. Cast off.
Sew in ends on wrong side.
Using oversewing, stitch up shoulder seams and then stitch in sleeve (see instructions for multi-coloured jumper opposite.
Sew up side and arm seams leaving ¾in (2cm) open at bottom of side seams. Press with a damp cloth.

Sleeve shaping
Cast off 4 stitches at the beginining of the next 2 rows, which leaves (44, 48, 52) stitches. Continue with pattern until (7, 8, 9) green stripes have been worked.

Neck shaping
Knit (11, 12, 13) stitches. Continue on these until 2 more green stripes have been worked. Cast off.
Cast off centre stitches (22, 24, 26). Knit on remaining (11, 12, 13) stitches until 2 green stripes have been worked. Cast off.

To make a button loop
Make a double loop with the yarn on the edge of the knitting or crochet.
The size should be just big enough to fit over the button (*fig 10a*).
Work over the loops made in buttonhole stitch (*fig 10b*). Fasten off.

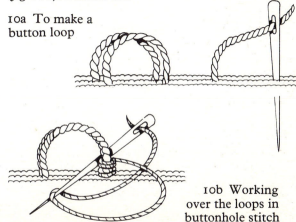

10a To make a button loop

10b Working over the loops in buttonhole stitch

71

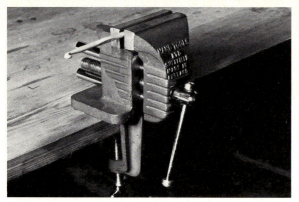

11 Position of crochet hook in vice

CROCHET

A crochet hook is placed in a vice with the hook facing towards you (*fig 11*). If you are using your right hand the hook should be pointing to the right and vice versa for the left hand. A Tunisian crochet hook, which is like a knitting needle with a crochet hook at one end, is most suitable because it is longer than the usual hook and so holds the work further from the vice, but an ordinary hook will do. It is a good idea to have your yarn in a bowl or box on the table to stop it from rolling onto the floor as you work. The advantage of crochet is that you have only one stitch to drop and if you do happen to make a mistake it is very easy to undo. When crocheting using two hands: the wool is usually held still in one hand and it is the hook that is manoevred. When using a vice this has to be reversed – as the hook is held still, the wool must be wound around it.

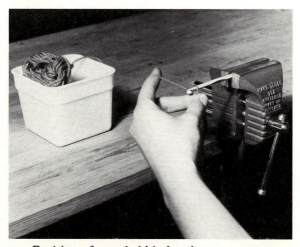

12a Position of yarn held in hand

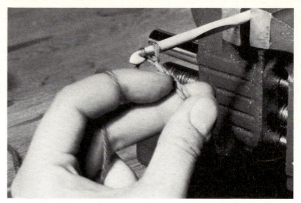

12b Making a chain

Stitches

Chain (abbreviation ch)
First make a slip loop and place it over the hook. Hold the stitch and short end of yarn with the thumb and second finger and have the working yarn over the index finger and through the rest of your hand, gripping it with your little finger (*fig 12a*). You may find this very awkward at first but persevere, as it will make crocheting easier in the long run. Using the index finger bring the working yarn from behind the hook over it and catch it in the hook (*fig 12b*). Then draw the chain on the hook over the yarn and off, thus forming the next chain; repeat.

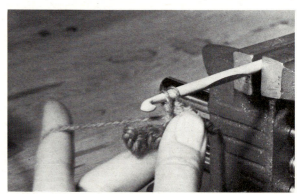

13 Two threads on the hook for dc

Double crochet (abbreviation dc)
Put the hook through the work and draw the working yarn through the work, making two threads on the hook (*fig 13*). Then bring the yarn over the hook from the back, catching it with the hook, draw through the two loops to complete the stitch.

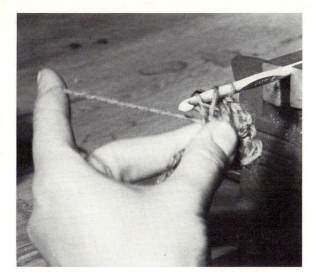

14a Three threads on the hook

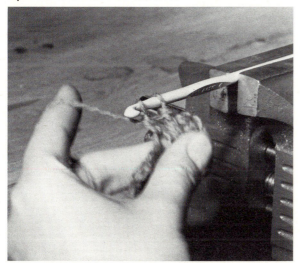

14b Leaving two threads on the hook

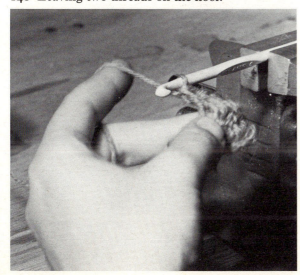

14c Treble forward

Treble (abbreviation tr)

Bring the yarn over the hook then insert hook through work and draw yarn through from back of the work thus making three threads on the hook (*fig 14a*). Bring the yarn over the hook and draw it through the first two threads, leaving two threads on hook (*fig 14b*). Bring the yarn over the hook and draw through the remaining two threads to form the treble (*fig 14c*).

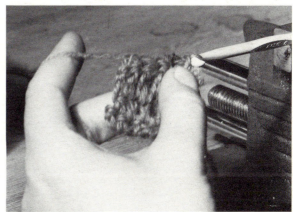

15 Slip stitch

Slip stitch (abbreviation ss)

Put hook through work, draw yarn through from the back straight through work and thread on hook (*fig 15*).

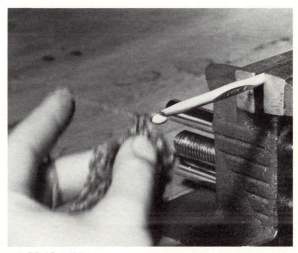

16 Half treble

Half treble (abbreviation htr)

Work as for treble when three threads are on hook, yarn over hook and straight through all three threads (*fig 16*).

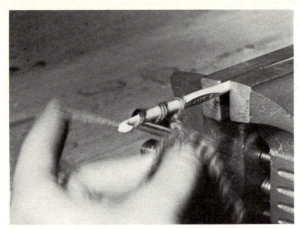

17a Yarn over hook twice for double treble

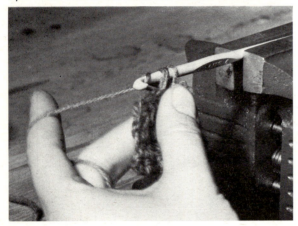

17b Working off double treble

Double treble (abbreviation dtr)
Yarn over hook twice, then put hook through work and draw through yarn from back of work, thus making four threads on hook. Yarn over hook, draw through two threads leaving three; yarn over hook, draw through two threads; yarn over hook, draw through two threads (*figs 17a and 17b*).

For the benefit of our American readers we give below the American equivalent of the English abbreviations of crochet terms used in our patterns.

English	American
ch	ss
dc	single or ch
tr	dc
htr	hdc
dtr	tr
trtr (triple treble)	dtr

Granny square or Afghan square
This is a good motif to start on as you are working into spaces rather than stitches.

The square is very attractive if each round is worked in a different colour, and this is also a good way of using up oddments. When joining a new colour, finish off the first colour by cutting the yarn and drawing the end through the chain on hook. Slip stitch the new colour to the place where you finished off the first colour and continue working as pattern.

You can also continue the square working more rounds; the groups of trebles between the corners will increase by one on each round. A

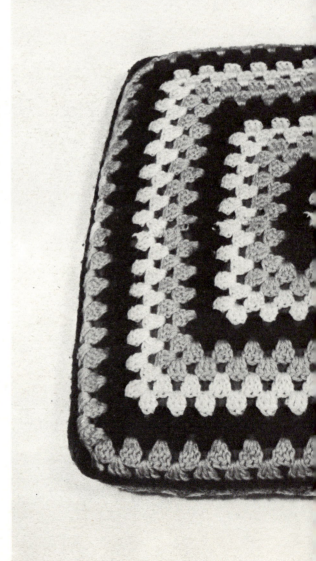

18 Cushion cover

large square can be used as a cushion cover (*18*) or shawl; the uses are endless.

Abbreviations: ch chain, tr treble, ss slip stitch, chsp chain space

Start circle

4 ch, ss to 1st chain to form a circle

Round 1

3 ch, 2 tr into circle. (3 ch, 3 tr) three times into circle. 3 ch, ss to 3rd of first 3 ch.

Round 2

3 ch, 2 tr into corner space under 3 ch. *1 ch (3 tr, 3 ch, 3 tr) into next 3 chsp. Repeat from * twice. 1 ch. 3 tr 3 ch into first corner space. ss to 3rd ch of 1st 3 ch.

Round 3

3 ch 2 tr into corner space under 3 ch. *1 ch 3 tr into next 1 chsp. 1 ch (3 tr, 3 ch, 3 tr) into corner space. Repeat from * twice. 1 ch 3 tr into 1 chsp. 3 tr 3 ch into first corner space. ss to 3rd of 1st 3 ch.

Round 4

3 ch, 3 tr into corner space below 3 ch. *(1 ch, 3 tr into next 1 chsp) twice. 3 tr, 3 ch, 3 tr into corner space. Repeat from * three times omitting final 3 tr. ss to 3rd of 1st 3 ch.

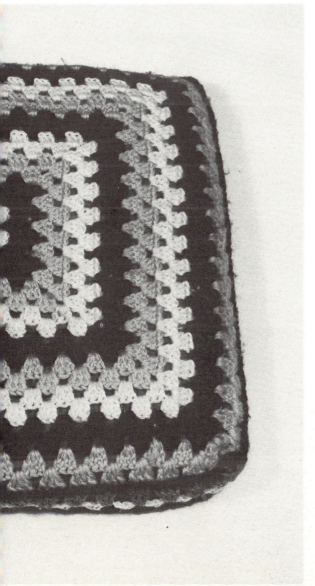

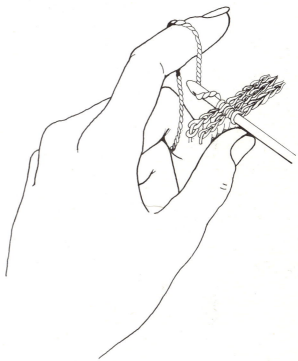

19 Joining crochet with slip stitch

Joining by crochet

Place the two pieces of work to be joined with right sides together and edges level with each other. Slip stitch the yarn to one end depending on which way you are working. Then place the hook through the first stitches of both pieces of work and slip stitch. Continue in this way into each stitch (*fig 19*). This gives a fairly flat seam.

By using the same method but working a double crochet instead of a slip stitch two pieces of work can be joined with more of a ridged seam. This can be quite effective if worked on the right side with a contrasting colour.

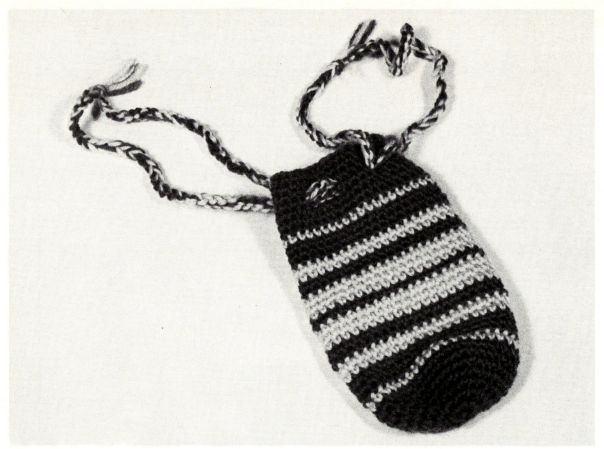

20a Crochet purse

Crochet Purse

Materials
Hermit Double Knitting 100% wool:
1 × 1 oz (or 25g) ball Almond (A), 1 × 1 oz (or 25g) ball Oatmeal (B)
No 3.00 crochet hook

Instructions
Using A: 4 ch ss to form ring.
Round 1
10 dc into ring, ss to first dc.
Round 2
2 dc into every st, ss to first dc (20 dc).
Round 3
(1 dc into first st, 2 dc into next st), repeat to end. ss to first dc (30 dc).
Round 4
(1 dc into each of next 2 sts, 2 dc in next st.), repeat to end. ss to first dc (40 dc).
Round 5
1 dc in every st, ss to first dc.

Rounds 6 and 7 as Round 5.
ss in colour B. Continue working in same st, as follows:
1 round B
3 rounds A
2 rounds B
2 rounds A
3 rounds B
1 round A
3 rounds B
2 rounds A
2 rounds B
3 rounds A
1 round B
3 rounds A
Using A only: next round (4 dc, 1 ch, miss 1 st).
Repeat to end. Three more rounds of dc. Cast off.
To make cord : Using two threads at once, one of each colour, make two lengths of chain 20in (50cm) long. Thread through holes made. Sew in ends (*figs 20b and 20c*).

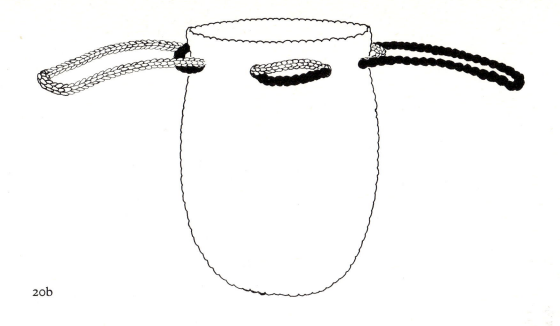

20b

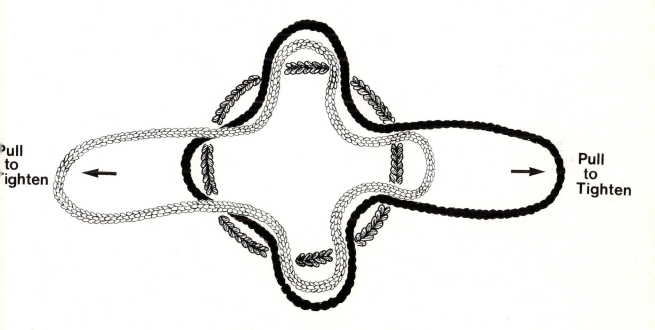

CROSS-SECTION OF PURSE

20c

Shawl

The shawl illustrated used the following materials, but any yarn could be used for this pattern, and it can also be any size.

Materials

Hermit brushed mohair/wool Double Knitting, 8 × 1oz (or 25g) balls
No 3.00 crochet hook

Instructions

Row 1
11 ch, 2 tr into 7th ch from hook, 1 ch miss 1 ch, 2 tr in next ch, miss 1 ch, 1 tr in last ch.
Row 2
4 ch, 1 tr in first chsp, 1 ch, 2 tr in same chsp, 1 ch, 2 tr in next space, 1 ch, 2 tr, 1 ch, 2 tr in last space. Turn.
Row 3
4 ch, 2 tr in first space, 1 ch, (2 tr 1 ch) in each space to end. 1 tr in top 4th ch of previous row.
Row 4
4 ch (1 tr, 1 ch, 2 tr) in first space, (1 ch, 2 tr) in each space to end. (1 ch, 2 tr, 1 ch, 2 tr) in the end 4 chsp.

Repeat Rows 3 and 4 until shawl is required size.

Keep one ball of wool for fringe. Cut length of 2 in (5 cm). Using three strands together, attach to the end of each row to form fringe. See p 18 for method of looping a fringe.

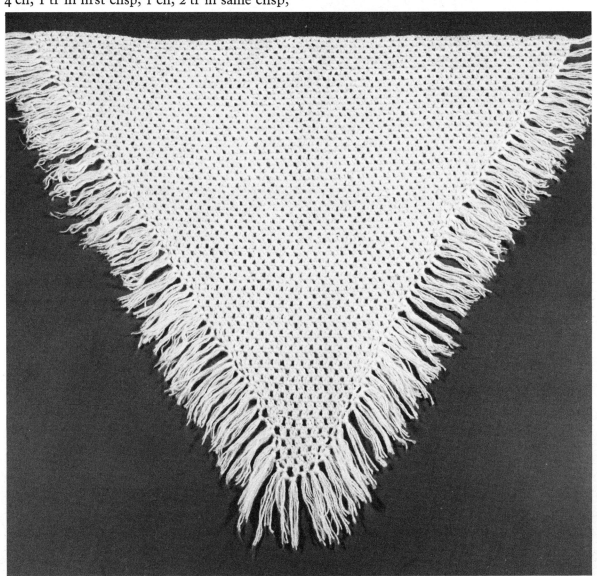

21 Shawl

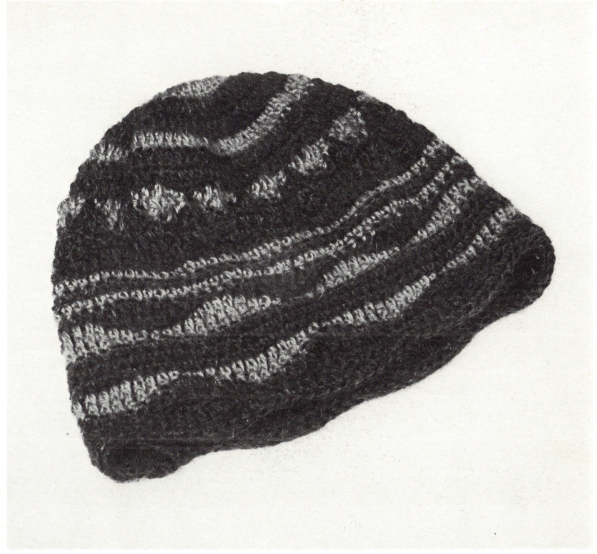

22 Hat

Hat

To fit average size head.

Materials

Patons Kismet wool, 6 × 1oz (or 3 × 50g) balls in Blue (B), Brown (BR) and Orange (O)
No 3.50 crochet hook

Instructions

Using O: 4 ch, ss to form ring.

Row 1

3 ch, 15 tr into ring, ss to 3rd of first 3 ch.

Row 2

3 ch, 1 tr in same place as 3 ch, 2 tr in every st. ss to 3rd of first 3 ch (34sts including 3 ch).

Row 3

Join in BR with ss. 3 ch (2 tr in next st, 1 tr in next). Repeat to end. ss to 3rd of 3 ch (51 sts).

Row 4

Join in B with ss. 3 ch, 1 tr *2 tr in next st, 1 tr in each of next 2 sts. Repeat from * to end. ss to 3rd of first 3 ch (68 sts).

Row 5

Join in O. 3 ch, 1 tr on each of next 2 sts, *2 tr in next st, 1 tr on each of next 3 sts. Repeat from * to end. ss to 3rd of first 3 ch (85 sts).

Row 6

Join in BR. 3 ch, 1 tr in every st, ss to join.

Row 7

Join in B. 3 ch 1 tr in every st, ss to join.

Row 8
Join in O. *1 htr in first tr, 1tr in 2nd tr, 1 dtr. 1 ch 1dtr in next tr, 1 tr in next tr, 1 htr in next tr. Miss 1 st, repeat from * to end, ss to htr.

Row 9
Join in BR. 3 ch, 1 dtr into same place as 3 ch, 1 tr in tr. *1 htr in 1 chsp, 1 tr in tr, 2 dtr in space between 2 htr. 1 tr in tr. Repeat from * to end. ss to 3rd of first 3 ch.

Row 10
ss along to first htr. Working into each st, * 1 htr 2 tr on next 2 sts. (1 dtr, 2 ch, 1 dtr) into next st, 2 dtr on next 2 sts, 2 tr on next 2 sts. Repeat from * to end. ss to first htr. Seven points made.

Row 11
Join in B. 4 ch, 1 dtr on each of next 2 sts. * 1 tr on each of next 2 sts. 1 htr, 1 dc into chsp. 1 htr on next st, 1 tr in each of next 2 sts. 5 dtr on next 5 sts. Repeat from * to end. Finish with 2 dtr. ss to 4th of first 4 ch.

Row 12
Join in O. 1 ch, 1 htr in every st. ss to 1 ch.

Row 13
Join in BR. Repeat Row 12.

Row 14
Join in O. Repeat Row 12.

Row 15
Join in B. 4 ch working in each st. 3 dtr * 2 tr, 1 htr, 1 dc, 2 tr, 5 dtr. Repeat from * to end. Ending with 1 dtr, ss to 4th of first 4 ch.

Row 16
Join in O. 1 ch * 1 dc, 1 htr, 2 tr, 5 dtr, 2tr, 1 htr. Repeat from * to end. ss to first dc.

Rows 17–19
Repeat Rows 12–14 with the colours BR, B, BR respectively.

Row 20
Join in O. * 1 htr, 1 dc, 1 htr, 2 tr, 5 dtr, 2 tr. Repeat from * to end. ss to first htr.

Row 21
Join in BR. 4 ch, 4 dtr, 2 tr, * 1 htr, 1 dc, 1 htr, 2 tr, 5 dtr, 2 tr. Repeat from * to end. ss to 4th of first 4 ch.

Row 23
2 ch 1 htr in every st. Cast off.
Sew in loose ends.
A simpler version of this hat can be made by working the first seven rows and then continuing in trebles until deep enough to fit. This could either be in stripes or all one colour.

Child's top

Size
Chest 20, 22, 24in (51, 55, 59cm)
Length 12, 13, 14in (29, 32, 35cm)

Materials
Wendy Double Knitting 100% wool (5, 5, 6) × 1oz (or 25g) Pilot Blue (A)
1 × 1oz (or 25g) Antique Jade (B)
1 × 1oz (or 25g) Grey (C)
No 3.50 crochet hook

Tension
10 tr and 6 rows to 2in (5cm)

Body
Make two the same, as follows:
Using A, make (58, 62, 66) ch.
Row 1

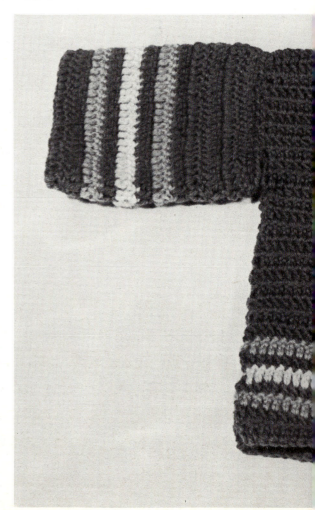

23 Child's top

1 tr into 4th ch from hook. 1 tr in every ch to end. (55, 59, 63) sts, including turning ch.

Row 2
3 ch (standing as first tr), tr to end of row. This forms the pattern.

Row 3
Using B

Row 4
Using A

Row 5
Using C

Row 6
Using A

Row 7
Using B
Then work (27, 31, 34) rows in A. Cast off.

Sleeves
Make two the same, as follows:
Using A, cast on (49, 53, 57) ch.

Row 1
1 tr in 4th ch from hook, tr to end (46, 50, 54).

Row 2
3 ch, 1 tr in every st.

Row 3
Using B

Row 4
Using A

Row 5
Using C

Row 6
Using A

Row 7
Using B
Then work (6, 8, 10) rows in A. Cast off.
Sew in ends and stitch up, using oversewing. Leave neck space open at centre ($5\frac{1}{2}$, $5\frac{1}{2}$, 6) in (or 14, 14, 15cm).
The seams can be crocheted together using either slip stitch or double crochet.

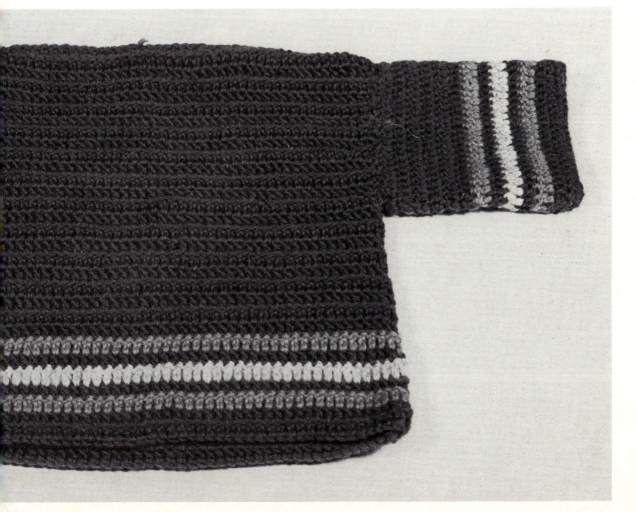

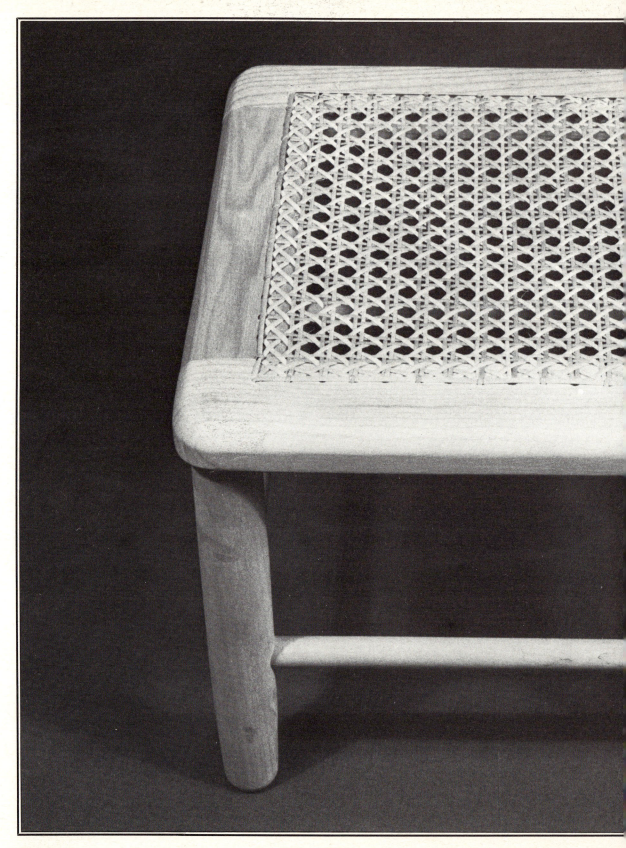

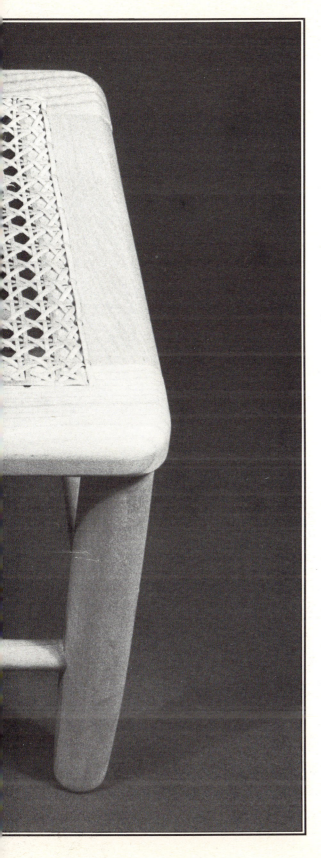

4 Chair Caning

The craft of caning chairs is extremely old, the earliest evidence of the technique dating back to The Ancient Egyptians. It was introduced into England in the seventeenth century. It was light, airy, inexpensive and decidedly preferable to the upholstery of the time, which was prone to maggots! Caned furniture has been in and out of fashion over the years since then but has never completely disappeared and is currently enjoying a considerable revival of popularity.

There are several patterns and numerous different shapes which can be worked. They vary in complexity but the actions used in working are the same. The scale is large enough to be worked by someone with imperfect eyesight. Each piece of cane is held in place by a peg as it is worked so it is not necessary to exert continuous effort and can therefore be worked by those with shaky hands provided there is some co-ordination. It can also be worked with one hand only.

Beside the traditional use of these techniques on chair seats and backs, for anyone interested and able to do woodwork as well it would be possible to make many other articles such as screens or shutters, a bedhead or table top.

MATERIALS

Cane

Cane is imported from south-east Asia. It is a
creeper which has a thorny outer bark under
which is a hard shiny surface which is used for
chair seating. It is stripped off, cut to reason-
able lengths, uniform widths (sized 0–6) and
sold in 9oz (or 250g) bundles. The inner pith of
the plant is processed to produce cane for
basket making but is also used sometimes for
pegs on chair seats.

Tools *(fig 1)*

A fine BODKIN is used for clearing a space in a
hole during the late stages when they become
blocked.
A pair of SCISSORS for trimming ends.
A KNIFE for cutting away an old cane seat and
also for trimming ends.
A CLEARER is used for clearing out the holes
when stripping an old chair ready for a new
seat.
A SHELL BODKIN can be used during the later
stages when the cane is interwoven. It is
essential for a one-handed worker.
PEGS are used to hold the cane in place during
the working of the seat. They can be made by
sharpening the end of a piece of No 15 centre
cane then cutting it off about 2in (5cm) long.
Alternatively plastic golf tees are also suitable
for the purpose.
A BOWL OF WARM WATER; all that is required in
preparation of the cane is to dip it briefly in
warm water to soften it.
A SMALL HAMMER is useful in conjunction with
the clearer and also for hammering in plugs
when the stool is complete.
PLUGS are used in finishing off a seat and are cut
from small pieces of centre cane.

A stool or chair

It is possible to buy small stools made for the
purpose with holes already drilled. These are
quite quick to do and suitable for a beginner as
the square shape is the easiest to do.
    There are plenty of old chairs around in junk
shops or antique shops in quite good condition
which only need recaning. Quite often a
plywood top has been nailed on to the chair
when the original caning has worn out.

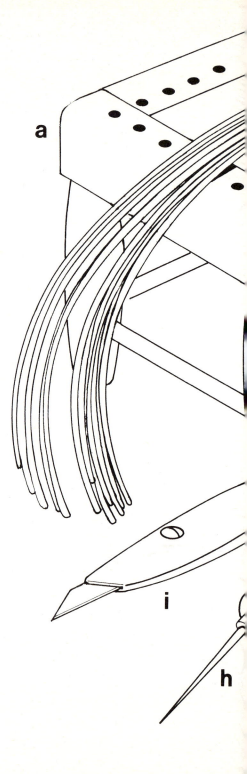

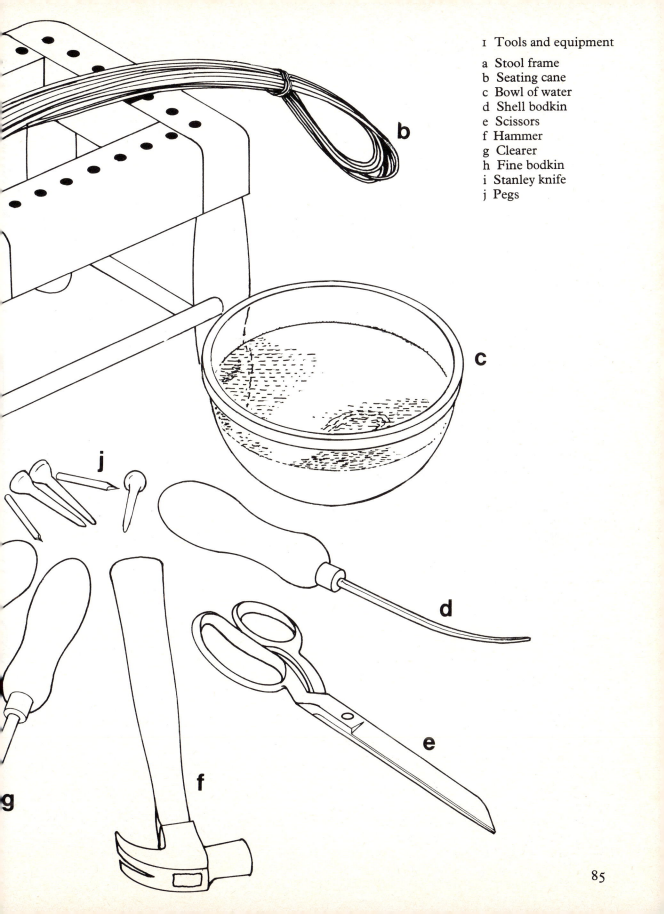

1 Tools and equipment

a Stool frame
b Seating cane
c Bowl of water
d Shell bodkin
e Scissors
f Hammer
g Clearer
h Fine bodkin
i Stanley knife
j Pegs

b

c

j

d

e

f

g

Preparing an old chair

• First, cut most of the cane away using a knife.
• Use the clearer and a hammer to clear the old plugs and remnants of cane from the holes (*fig 2*).
• Clean up the chair using turpentine or white spirit on a piece of rag. You may need to use wire wool on any awkward corners.
• The chair can then be finished with polish, varnish or paint.

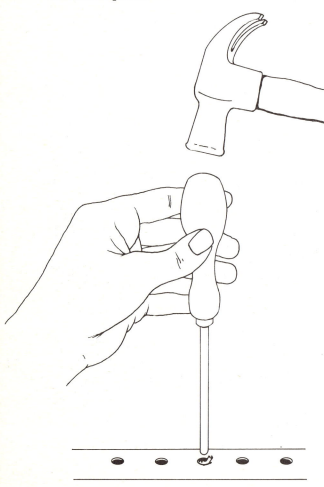

2 Using the clearer to remove the remains of an old seat

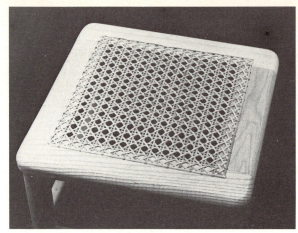

3 Caned stool with beading

HOW TO CANE A SQUARE STOOL
Using the 6 stage traditional pattern

Materials
A stool
No 2 and No 4 seating cane
Tools (*fig 1*)
Polyurethane varnish (available in gloss, matt or satin finish)
Turpentine or white spirit
Rags
Sandpaper

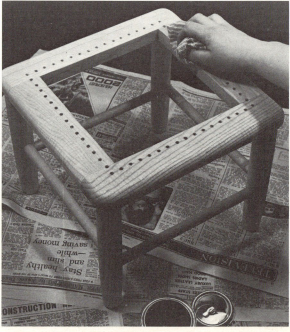

4 Varnishing the stool using a rag

Sand down any roughness on the stool. Using a rag (to avoid brush marks) work the varnish over the stool so the whole stool is covered (*fig 4*). Leave to dry according to instructions on the tin.

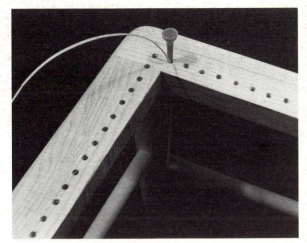

5 Pegging the first piece of cane

STAGE 1 First setting (No 2 cane)

The settings go from the back to the front of the seat and the weavings go from side to side. It will help to mark one foot rail of the stool with a piece of string and call that the front.

Remove a piece of cane from the bundle. The easiest way to do this is to pull one strand from the looped end. Dip it briefly in bowl of warm water to soften it.

Place one end into the second hole from the left at the back so it protrudes underneath about 3 in (8 cm) and place a peg in to hold it (*fig 5*). Bring the other end of the cane towards the front and thread it through the corresponding opposite hole and peg. The shiny side should be uppermost. It is not necessary to pull tightly but the cane should be firm. For a one-handed worker it is possible to hold the cane down with a weight while placing the peg in the hole, but if possible it is quicker to grip the cane between the knees.

Underneath the stool turn the cane to the right and thread up through the next hole so that the shiny side is showing underneath and peg from the top (*fig 6*). The weight can also be used here but it can be quicker to use your teeth. Repeat this back and forward across the stool, removing all but the first and last pegs as you go (*fig 7*).

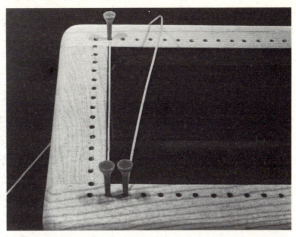

6 Continuing the first setting

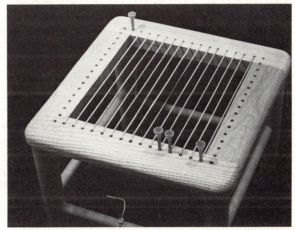

7 First setting completed

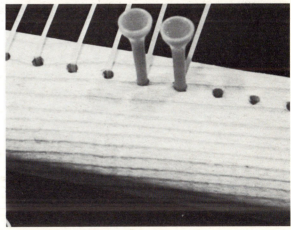

8 Joining a new piece of cane

To join a new piece of cane
Peg the end of the first piece, making sure the remaining end is at least 3 in (8 cm) long. Peg a new piece in the next hole leaving an end of 3 in (8 cm) and continue (*fig 8*).

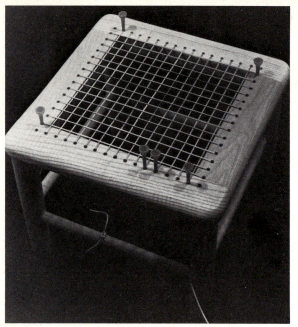

9 First weaving

10 Second setting

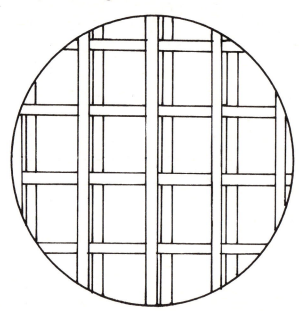

STAGE 2 First weaving (No 2 cane)
Work the first weaving like the first setting, but taking the cane from side to side across the stool and laying it on top of the first setting (*fig 9*).

STAGE 3 Second setting (No 2 cane)
The second setting is worked into the same holes as the first setting but the cane is placed slightly to the left and is laid on top of the first weaving (*fig 10*). Try to work so that the spaces between the holes underneath the stool are all covered equally; do not build up layers on alternate spaces.

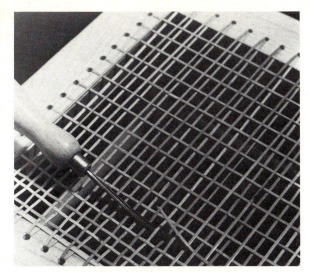

11a Using the shell bodkin

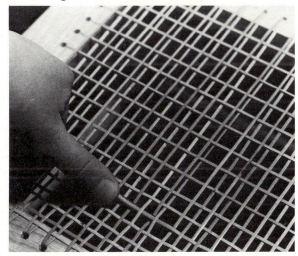

11b Using the shell bodkin

The second weaving is woven under and over the settings, the opposite way to the first weaving. It is placed in the same holes but towards the back of the stool (*fig 12*).

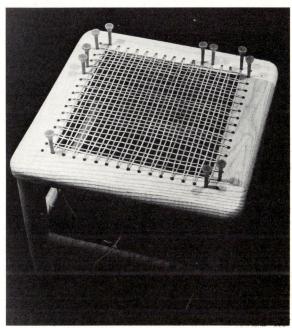

12 Second weaving

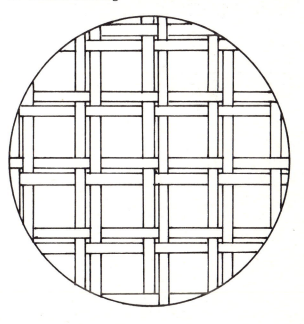

STAGE 4 Second weaving (No 2 cane)

As this and succeeding stages are actually interwoven, it is necessary to work with the grain otherwise any rough pieces can catch and split. To find the grain when selecting a new piece of cane, run the thumb nail along the cane on the shiny side first one way and then the other. One way will catch more than the other; weave the cane in its smoother direction. It is helpful to cut the cane to a point from this stage onwards.

The SHELL BODKIN can be used at this stage. Weave it under and over four threads. Push the pointed end of the cane into the shell of the bodkin, right through the four threads, grip with the thumb and pull through completely as the bodkin is pulled out (*figs 11a, 11b*).

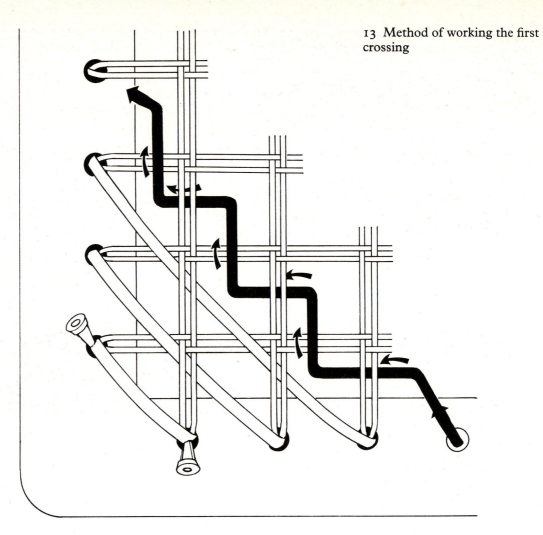

13 Method of working the first crossing

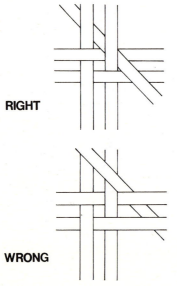

RIGHT

WRONG

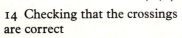

14 Checking that the crossings are correct

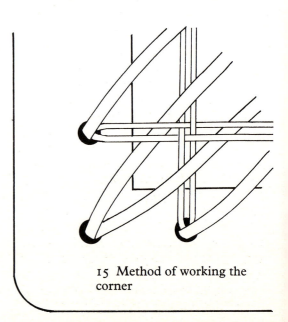

15 Method of working the corner

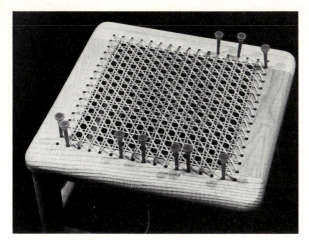

16 First crossing

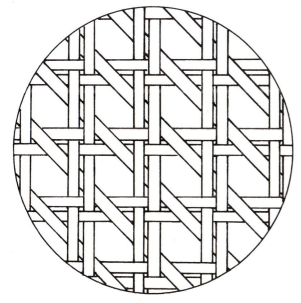

STAGE 6 Second crossing (No 4 cane)
Starting at the front right-hand corner of the stool, work as for the first crossing but in the opposite direction, ie, bottom right to top left, going under the weavings and over the settings (*fig 17*). Remember to work twice in the corners at the halfway point.

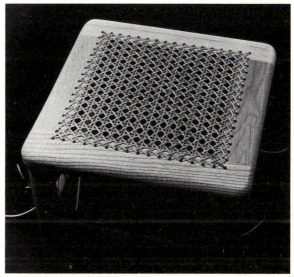

17 Second crossing

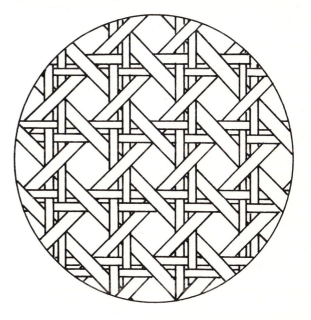

STAGE 5 First crossing (No 4 cane)
As by this time the holes are becoming full it may be necessary to clear a space for the next piece of cane by using a fine bodkin.

The first crossing starts on the first hole on the left side of the stool (not the corner hole) and runs down to the first hole on the left end of the front of the stool. Although the result is a diagonal the motion used in working is a stepping action, going under the settings and over the weavings (*fig 13*). It is important to get the crossings going the correct way. They should slip between the setting and weaving when pulled through and not bite into the corners (*fig 14*).

At the halfway point it is necessary to go twice into the corner holes (*fig 15*).

Finishing off

Turn the stool upside down and work from underneath. Any holes that have one end in can be tied off in one of two ways (*figs 18a, 18b*). Any holes that have two ends in can be tied off by taking one end to the right and one to the left. If there are more than two ends in any hole, tying off would be too messy, so you must plug or peg these holes.

Cut a plug from a piece of centre cane, no longer than the depth of the stool top, and trim it to a point. It must be thick enough to fit tightly in the hole. Hammer it into place, if necessary using the clearer to ensure that the peg does not jut up above the surface of the stool.

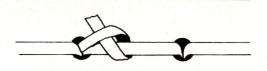

18a Method of tying off

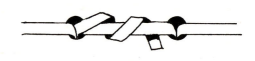

18b Method of tying off

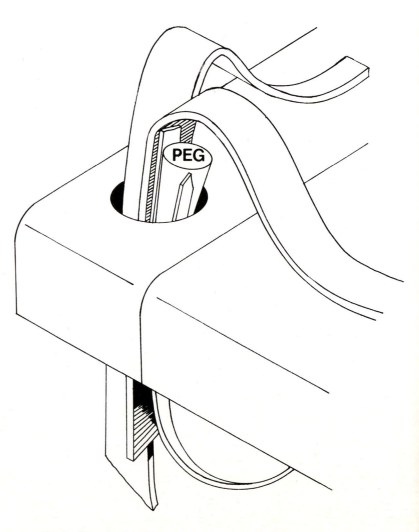

19a Beginning the beading

USING BEADING TO FINISH OFF

Beading is a method of laying a length of thick cane round the edge of the finished seat to cover up all the holes. It is held in place by a piece of fine cane (couching thread).

All the ends must be finished off first. If it is necessary to peg any of the holes it must be alternate holes only. Any ends in other holes that need to be pegged can be carried across and taken upwards into a hole that can be pegged.

You need No 6 seating cane for the beading and No 2 for the couching thread.

Insert one piece of No 6 into the front left-hand corner hole with an end protruding below and lay it along the left side of the stool, shiny side uppermost. Insert a second piece with the shiny side down on top of the first piece. Push the end of a length of No 2 (couching thread) upwards through the same hole and plug all three in place (*figs 19a and 19b*). Trim the end of the No 2 and fold the second piece of No 6 down along the front of the stool.

Carry the couching thread underneath the front of the stool and up the second hole (it will probably be necessary to use a bodkin). Take the thread over the beading and down the same hole, ensuring that the beading covers the hole exactly (*fig 20*). Make sure the shiny side of the couching thread is alway the side showing. Continue along the front, couching through every alternate hole until you reach the right-hand corner. The couching thread must be long enough to reach a corner when it is worked, so that any joins occur at the corners where they can be plugged in place with the beading. Take the beading down the corner hole and place a new piece down the same hole. Fold the new piece back over the old piece (the underneath side of the new piece will be showing) and plug the hole. Take the new piece along the right-hand side of the stool and continuing the couching work all the way round the stool.

The top left-hand corner may need plugging; just finish the ends off underneath. If it is necessary you must plug upwards from underneath the seat.

Finally continue the couching thread along the left-hand side of the stool and fasten off underneath at the end.

If you are working on a curved or round seat you will find that the beading will stretch enough to make a neat curve to fit.

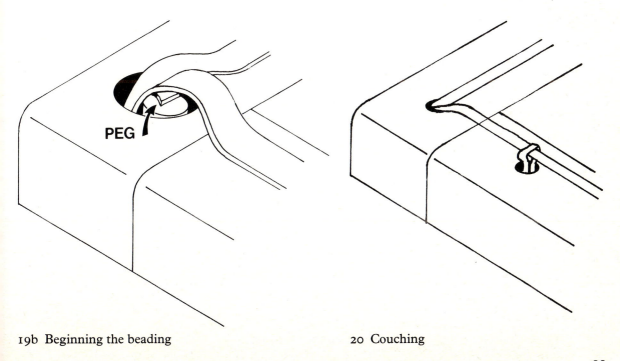

PEG

19b Beginning the beading

20 Couching

WORKING OTHER SHAPES

are worked as normal.

Rectangular
Work as for square.

Concave (fig 21)
Work the first stage, then the third stage, across from curved edge to curved edge. Then, work the second stage, which will need to be interwoven like the fourth stage. The crossings

Curved, bow- or wide-fronted shapes
Start the first stage in the centre of the seat, working outwards to either side (fig 22). When you reach the shaping at the sides or front it will not be necessary to use every hole (fig 23). Choose the holes that will allow the cane to lie parallel to the previous row. Choosing the holes in this way will be necessary for each succeeding stage as well.

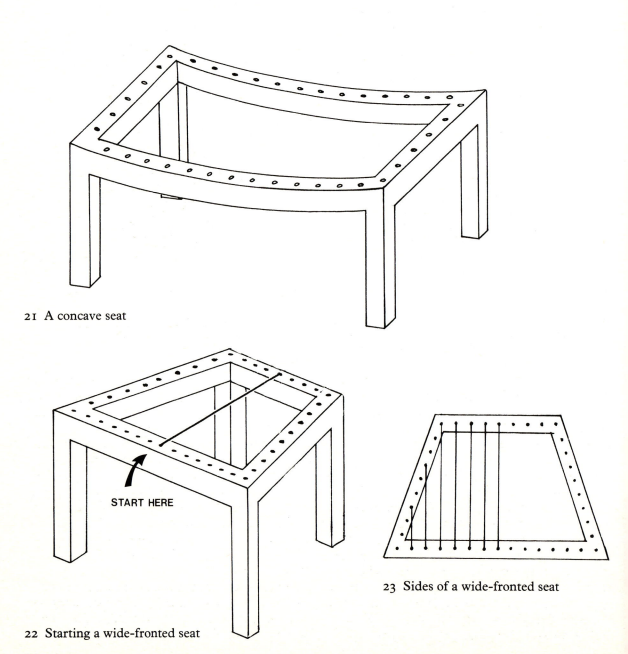

21 A concave seat

START HERE

22 Starting a wide-fronted seat

23 Sides of a wide-fronted seat

Circular

A plain circular seat is worked like the other curved shapes (see above).

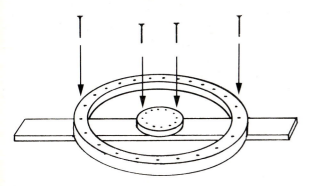

24 Nailing a circular back down before starting

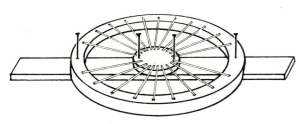

25 Beginning a circular back with stages 1 and 3

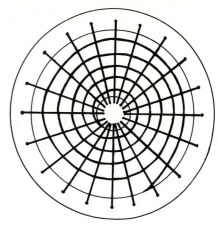

26a Spiral method of working stages 2 and 4

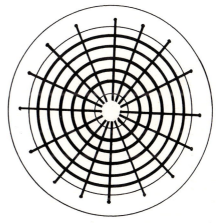

26b Circular method of working stages 2 and 4

Circular with a central boss

Chair backs are often worked in this way. You will need a piece of wood wider than the chair back. Using two of the holes in the chair, nail the wood across the back. Place the boss in the centre and nail it through two of its holes to the piece of wood. This will hold it in place until the first round is worked (*fig 24*).

Work stages 1 and 3 together from the outside edge to the inner boss. Work as much of these two stages as possible above and below the piece of wood (*fig 25*). Then remove the wood in order to complete the round.

Stages 2 and 4 are then worked together by one of two methods, either as a spiral (*fig 26a*) or as complete circles (*fig 26b*). With the circular method, each circle must be cut to length first and is complete in itself. The cane will stretch sufficiently to curve into a circle.

The crossings are worked normally.

HINTS ON WORKING

Blind holes

Sometimes a chair will have corner holes directly above the legs which cannot be drilled right through; these are blind holes. Some chairs consist entirely of blind holes.

The procedure for these is to cut the lengths of cane the right size to reach the bottom of the holes and glue in position with wood glue. Use plastic golf tees as pegs to hold the cane in position until the glue dries. The wood glue will not affect the plastic tees which can be removed easily when the glue has set.

Double caning

On some chair backs the caning is worked both on the inside and outside. The two sides are worked together with the same cane. This can be very complicated to do.

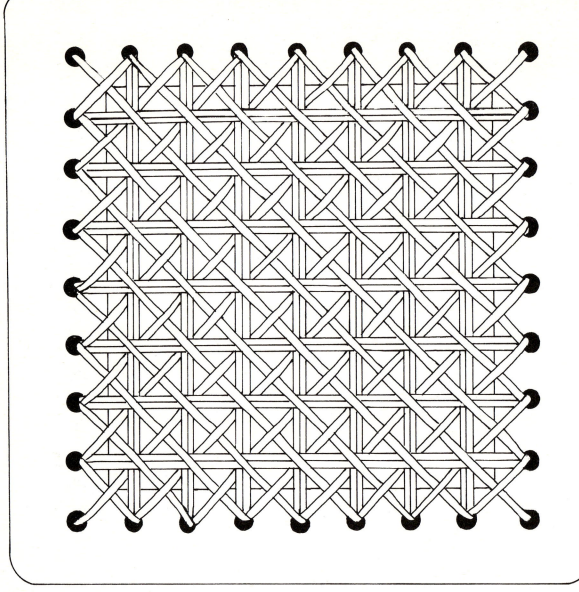

OTHER PATTERNS FOR CANING

27 Double Victoria pattern:
Double setting of No 2 cane
Double weaving of No 2 cane
2 crossings of No 3 cane

There are other patterns besides the 6 stage traditional pattern, such as the Double Victoria (*fig 27*) and the 4 way standard (*fig 28*).

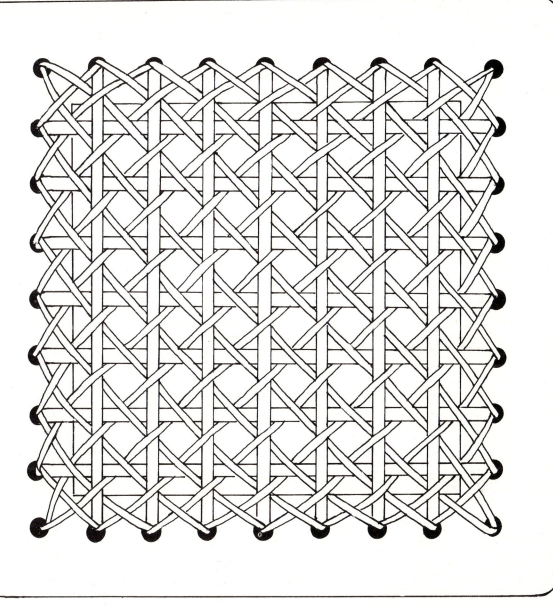

28 4 way standard pattern:
1 setting of No 4 cane
1 weaving of No 4 cane
2 crossings of No 3 cane

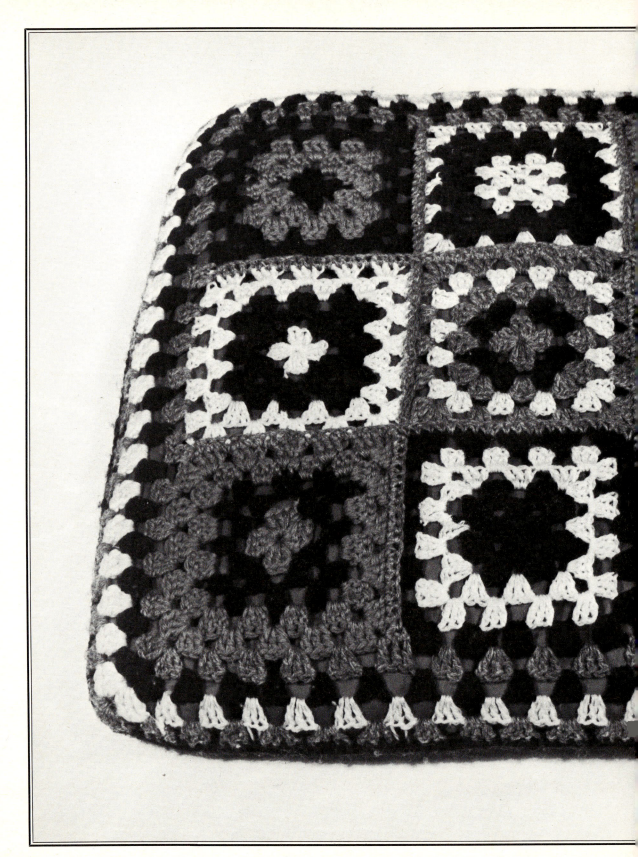

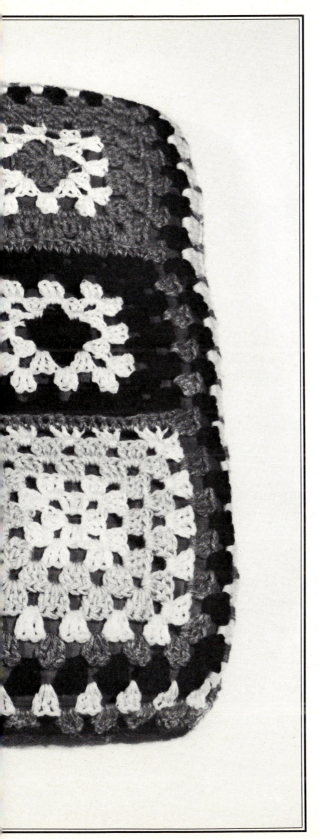

5 Coils, Circles and Squares

In this chapter we try to show how, with a small range of techniques and materials, basic units can be made which when joined together can form a variety of useful and decorative articles. The units we show how to make are :
Coiled work using French knitting tubes and plaited lengths of various materials
Circles cut from material or crocheted
Squares knitted or crocheted in wool (for techniques see chapter 3, Knitting and Crochet)

As a general rule the larger the scale worked on, the easier the craft becomes. Thus someone with poor sight might be able to manage French knitting with rug wool but not with crochet cotton. The materials given here are simply examples and we would suggest experimenting with different materials and yarns to find those which suit your own needs best. The crafts described here should be suitable for people with a varying degree of disability in their sight and grip.

EQUIPMENT

Sewing needles
Can be of a more substantial size than usual if that makes them easier to handle, and a large eye makes threading easier. Self-threading needles are also available. It can be helpful to use a double thread knotted together if the needle comes unthreaded easily (*fig 22, p 15*). A bodkin or large tapestry needle is useful for threading elastic.

A board with a hook
It is used for plaiting. If you buy the board at your local DIY supplier, ask the shopkeeper to screw the hook in for you.

A French knitting pin
(*fig 1*)

MATERIALS

A selection of knitting yarns, rug wool, raffia and Nytrim.
An assortment of fabrics, old or new.

COILED WORK TECHNIQUES

French knitting
French knitting is probably familiar to most people as a childhood pastime, using cotton reels to make reins. In the north east of Scotland fishermen's corks are used and it is known as 'catties' tails'. Cotton reels, alas, are no longer made of wood but plastic, so they are no longer suitable, but if you ask around you may find some old wooden ones. Otherwise you need to have a round knitting pin especially made (*fig 1*). This is suitable for some one who has poor or very little sight, lack of strong grip or unsteadiness. To work using one hand only a knitting pin with a stem (*fig 2*) can be used by holding it in a vice.

To thread a knitting pin
Push the end of the yarn through the centre hole leaving a tail, about 4 in (10 cm) long. Then wind the yarn round the first pin in a clockwise

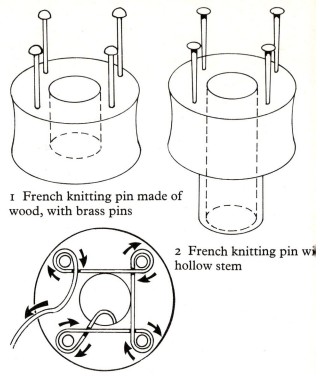

1 French knitting pin made of wood, with brass pins

2 French knitting pin wi hollow stem

3 Threading a knitting pin (arrow heads show direction of yarr

direction. Repeat this round the other three pins (*fig 3*).

To work
Hold the yarn firmly in front of the first pin and using either a crochet hook or large rug needle, hook the stitch on the pin over the yarn and the pin. Now give the tail of the yarn a good pull. Working anti-clockwise, repeat on each pin in turn. Continue working in this way until the required length of tube is made.

To join another colour
When joining another piece of yarn either of the same or a different colour, leave an end of about 2 in (5 cm). Tie the end of the new yarn to the old, as close as possible to the previous stitch. Poke the ends down into the tube of knitting and continue working with the new piece.

To cast off
Cut the working yarn and thread it through all four stitches on the knitting pin. Then take all the stitches off the pin and pull tight.

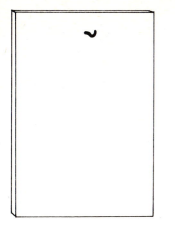

4 Board for plaiting with hook

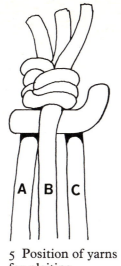

A B C

5 Position of yarns for plaiting

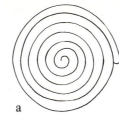

6 Coiled shapes made from either plaited lengths or French knitting lengths:
a Circle
b Oval
c Triangle
d Square
e Two triangles form base for diamond shape
f Two squares form base for oblong shape

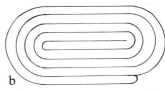

a

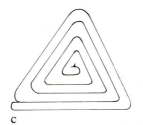

b

c

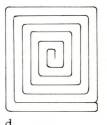

d

Plaiting

A plait can be worked in a variety of materials: raffia, wool, rags, Nytrim or anything that is long and pliable. It is a good idea to work on a piece of chip board 12 in × 20 in (30 cm × 50 cm) with a hook screwed in one end of it (*fig 4*). It should be quite heavy so that when the plait is pulled on, it will not shift off the table. As with French knitting, poor sight, lack of grip or unsteadiness should not be a hindrance, nor having only one hand or a lack of mobility. Also the larger the scale of plait, the easier it will be

To plait with yarn

You need three lengths of yarn; knot them together at one end. Hook this knot onto the hook on the board and spread out the yarns, calling them, A, B and C respectively from left to right (*fig 5*). Take A, the left-hand strand, over B to lie in the centre between B and C. Then take C, which is on the right, over A to lie in the centre between B and A. Continue in this way alternating between the left and right outside strands, trying to have an even pull on each strand which will give a balanced tension to the plait.

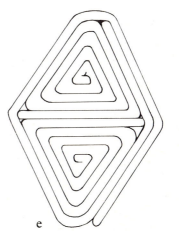

e

COILED WORK

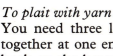

Tubes of french knitting and lengths of plaiting can be tightly coiled and stitched on the back to make a variety of articles. Circles, ovals, triangles, squares and oblongs are some different shapes that can be made (*fig 6*).

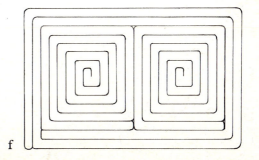

f

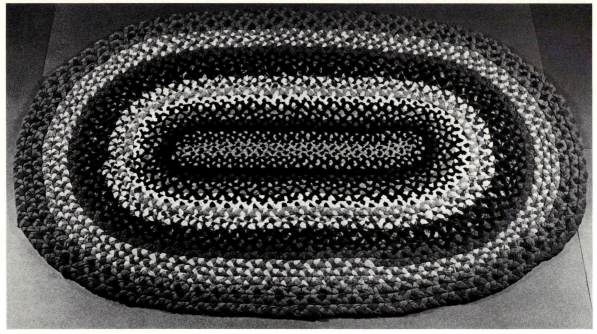

7 Plaited oval-shaped rag rug

Plaited oval-shaped rag rug

To plait with strips of material the strips should be of more or less the same weight of material. Natural fibres like cotton are easier to work with than man-made knitted fabrics, as the latter tend to stretch and pull out of shape.

Cut strips of material on the straight grain about 2 in (5 cm) wide and as long as the piece of material allows. Old curtains are ideal as you get a good length, but do not use material that is so old that it is rotten and splits easily.

Take three strips and knot them together firmly as close to the end as possible. Hook them to the board by the knot and start plaiting, keeping the raw edges rolled slightly under so that they do not show on the top of the plait.

When joining on a new piece place the new strip at right angles to the old and tack very firmly on the diagonal (*fig 8*).

If sewing is too difficult then a fabric glue such as Copydex can be used to stick the two ends together.

Continue plaiting until 1 yd (or 1 m) length is reached. You will need to keep unhooking the plait from the board and moving it up so that you can keep the same tension (*fig 9*).

On the wrong side fold the plait at about 12 in (30 cm) and using a strong thread, ladder stitch the folded plait together (*fig 10*).

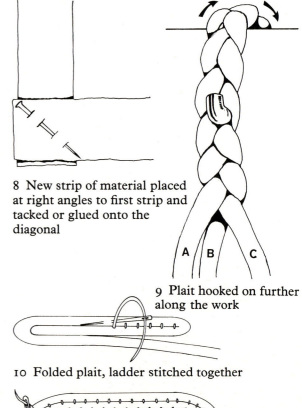

8 New strip of material placed at right angles to first strip and tacked or glued onto the diagonal

9 Plait hooked on further along the work

10 Folded plait, ladder stitched together

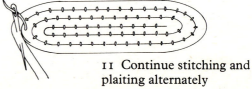

11 Continue stitching and plaiting alternately

Continue coiling the plait round and stitching it together (*fig 11*).

It is best to plait a length of about 1yd (or 1m) and then stitch it up rather than do great lengths of plaiting, so that the mat is formed as you go. Always lie the mat on a flat surface when stitching so that it does not buckle or pull out of shape.

Continue in this way until the mat is the required size.

Using colour

The three strands can be either all the same colour, which as expected gives a solid block of colour, or if each strand is a different colour you get a speckled effect. When changing from one solid colour to another you can lead the new colour in, gradually changing one strand first, then the second and finally the third. This would be over a length of about 3yds (or 3m), giving a shading effect.

Backing

A backing should be stitched onto the underside of the rug. Use hessian or any other strong fabric. Cut the backing out about $1\frac{3}{4}$in (4cm) larger than the rug all round. Fold the turning allowance under so that it is slightly smaller than the rug and ladder stitch the edge. For extra strength, iron-on or self-sticking carpet tape can be stuck round the edge.

French knitting round rug

For this rug you need a French knitting pin with a hole in the centre large enough to work with rug wool. Use odd balls of 6-ply rug wool

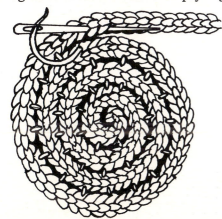

12 Coiling and stitching a French knitting tube; keep the same line of stitching showing all the time to prevent twisting

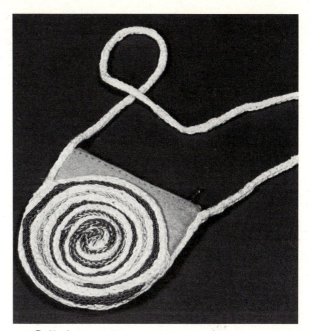

13 Coiled purse

in a variety of colours. Make about 1yd (or 1m) of knitting tube, then coil the tube round tightly. Working out from the centre, using the same colour, ladder stitch the tube together. It is important not to let the tube twist as it is inclined to do, so work on a flat surface and keep the ladder stitching through one line of stitching on the tube (*fig 12*). Continue working in this way, making a length of tube and then stitching it up, until the required size is reached. Stitch on a backing as for the plaited rug.

Coiled purse (*13*)

This can be made from either a French knitting tube or a plaited length. It is better to use a finer thread for making the knitting tube; crochet cotton worked on a cotton reel pin is ideal. If using plaiting, then plait with fine cotton material. Make two circular coiled pieces about 5in (12 cm) in diameter.

Cut two pieces of felt the same size as the coiled pieces and stitch onto the back of them. These will act as a lining for the purse and also strengthen the coiled work.

With right sides together ladder stitch the two pieces together leaving an opening at the top (*fig 14*). This opening can either be fastened with a couple of press-studs or a small zip can be stitched in by hand.

Make a length of knitting tube to fit round and hide the seam; stitch this on. If it is to be a body purse make this length of tube long enough to act as the strap as well (*fig 15*).

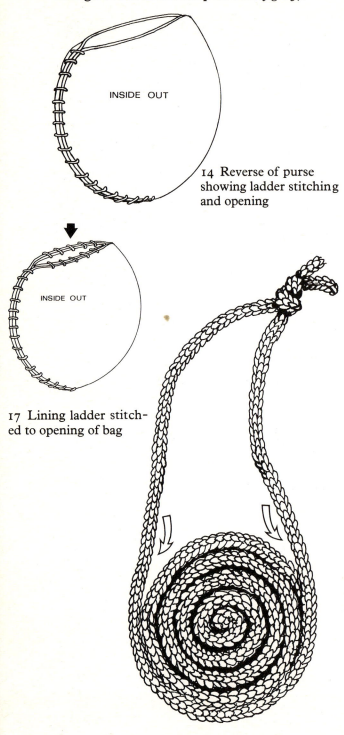

14 Reverse of purse showing ladder stitching and opening

17 Lining ladder stitched to opening of bag

15 Attaching the strap for a body purse

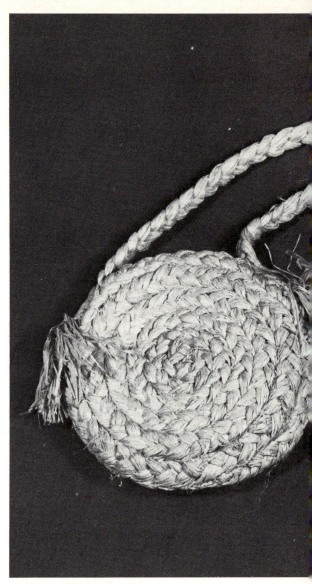

16 Coiled shoulder bag

Coiled shoulder bag

Again this can be made from either a French knitting tube or a plaited length. Double knitting wool would be suitable for French knitting. Raffia or Nytrim would be ideal for plaiting. As for the purse, make two circular coiled pieces about 8in (20cm) in diameter for a small bag, or about 12in (30cm) for a larger one.

With right sides together, ladder stitch the two pieces together leaving an opening at the top.

Cut out two circles slightly larger than the coiled ones in lining material. Stitch them round leaving the same opening at the top.

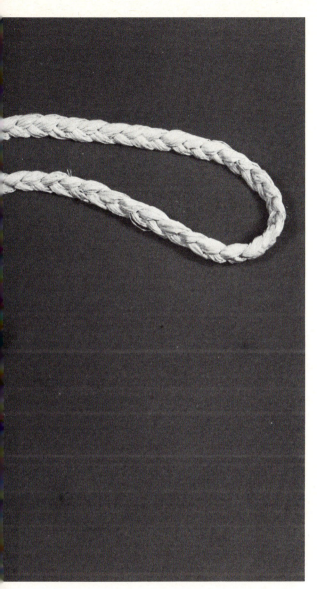

TECHNIQUES FOR MAKING CIRCLES

Material rosettes
This is a good way of using up scraps of material. You need to make a cardboard circle or template to draw round; this should be of fairly stiff cardboard with a diameter of about $5\frac{1}{2}$in (13 cm). Place the cardboard circle on the material and draw round it with a felt-tip or ballpoint pen. Then cut round the line drawn. It is best to draw a few circles and then cut them all out. Try and fit then onto the material so as to make the most ecomonic use of space.

Using the sewing cotton double with a knot in the end, gather round the edge of the circle about $\frac{1}{4}$in (5 mm) from the edge (*fig 18*). The stitches do not need to be particularly small, but try and keep them even.

When complete, gather up the circle tightly and overstitch a couple of times to secure (*fig 19*). Make plenty of these rosettes so that you have a good selection to choose from when making the various articles.

Crochet circle
For abbreviations and instructions on how to use a vice if one-handed, see chapter 3, Knitting and Crochet.
Using scraps of double knitting wool:
4 ch ss to form a circle. 3 ch, 15tr into ring. ss to 3rd of first 3 ch. Cast off. Darn in the two ends.

With the raw edges of the lining turned inside, slip the coiled bag (still inside out) into the lining and ladder stitch round the top (*fig 17*).

Make a length of plaiting or knitting tube long enough to form a handle and to go round the bottom of the bag. Turn the bag the right way out and stitch the handle on round the seam, as for the body purse.

Table mats
Table mats can be made up from any of the coiled shapes, made from either plaiting or French knitting tubes. A piece of felt, slightly smaller than the piece of coiled work, should be stuck on the back with a fabric glue.

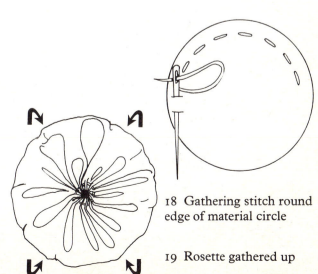

18 Gathering stitch round edge of material circle

19 Rosette gathered up

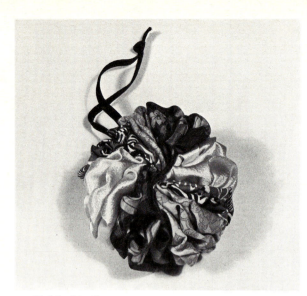

20 Babies' ball

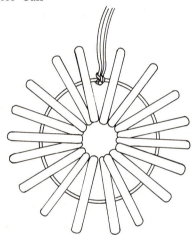

21 Rosettes pulled up tightly to
form a ball

USING CIRCLES

Babies' ball (20)

Use either crochet circles or material rosettes.

Use narrow elastic, with a bodkin that has a sharp point if you are using material rosettes.

Thread on about 40 circles. If the rosettes are made of thin fabric then you may need more than this number, or less if they are made of thick fabric.

Tie the ends of elastic together tightly leaving a long end to hang the ball by (fig 21).

This makes an ideal first toy for a baby. Several can be made to string across a pram or cot.

Caterpillar (22)

Onto narrow elastic, thread enough circles to fit tightly and measure 8in (20cm). Knot and stitch the elastic at both ends so that the circles cannot come off.

To make a head cut a large circle of plain material 6½in (16cm) in diameter. Gather round the edge in the same way as you make the rosettes but as you pull it up, stuff with some toy filling (see p 30). When pulled up stitch firmly to stop the stuffing coming out. Stitch this to one end of the length of circles. Cut out felt eyes and mouth and glue on (fig 23).

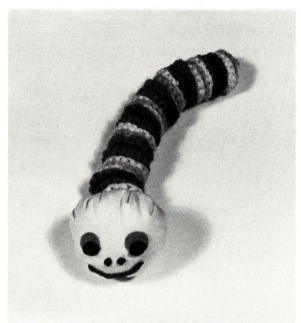

22 Caterpillar

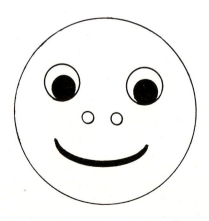

23 Caterpillar's face

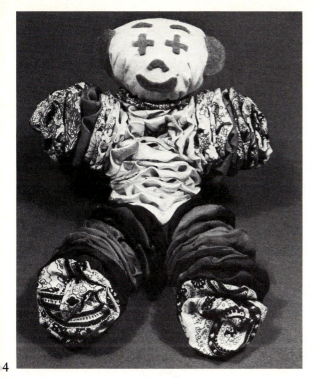

4

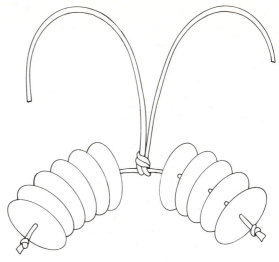

25 Threading and tying the
elastic for the clown's legs

Clown

Thread enough circles on a piece of narrow
elastic to make a length of 9½in (24cm). Knot or
stitch (or both) at both ends of the elastic. Find
the middle of this by counting the circles, loop
another piece of elastic around the middle and
tie (fig 25). This second piece of elastic needs to
be at least 14in (35cm) long and it should be
tied at the half-way point.

Thread this double through some more
circles making a 3¼in (8cm) length. This
forms the body while the first piece forms the
two legs. Now separate the elastic that you have
used double and thread each piece with enough
circles to make them each 3in (7cm) in length,
to form the arms. Tie another piece of elastic
round the division for the arms using it double
and thread on a few more circles to make the
neck (fig 26). Knot or stitch (or both) the ends of
the arms and the neck.

To make the head cut out a large circle of
white or pink plain fabric 7in (18cm) in
diameter. Stitch, gather and stuff as for
caterpillar's head. Now stitch this firmly to the
neck and stick on eyes, ears, nose and mouth
from felt (fig 27).

Four small silver bells can be stitched on the
arms and feet as an added attraction.

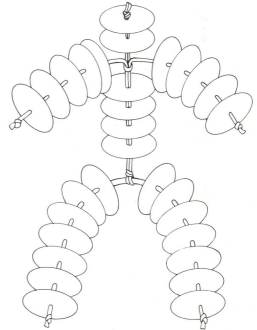

26 Joining and threading arms
and body to legs

27 Features of clown's face, cut
out from felt and glued on to
head

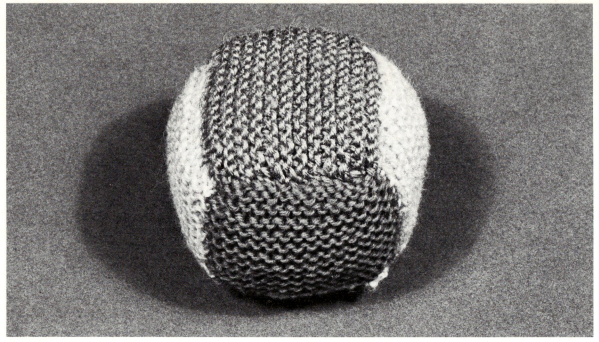

28 Soft play-brick

SQUARES

Making knitted and crochet squares are traditional occupations associated with elderly and disabled people. They make lovely gay blankets and knee rugs when stitched together. Here we have a few different ideas for making up the squares. For techniques see chapter 3, Knitting and Crochet.

The play bricks, bag on plywood handles and cushion cover could also be made with material squares, back stitched together. It is best to stitch them into strips and then stitch the strips together.

Soft play-bricks *(28)*
Knit six squares the same size in bright-coloured double knitting wool, each one a different colour.

Stitch together on the wrong side (*fig 29*). Before stitching the final side, turn the right side out and stuff firmly with some toy filling (see p 30). Ladder stitch the final sides together.

It would probably be best to make a set of 10 the same size.

The squares can be any size from 2 in × 2 in (5 cm × 5 cm) to 20 in × 20 in (50 cm × 50 cm)

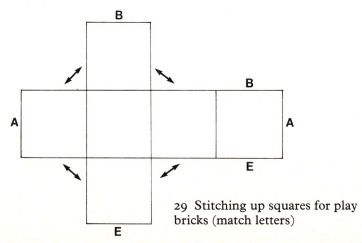

29 Stitching up squares for play bricks (match letters)

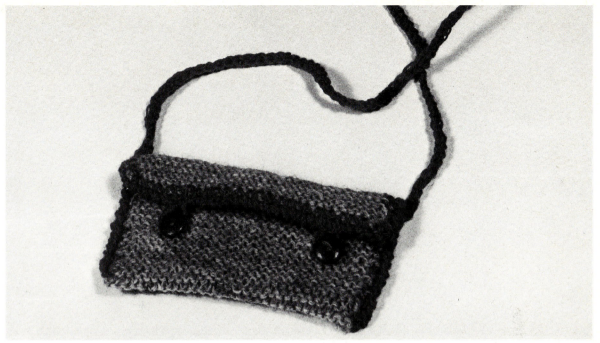

30 Purse

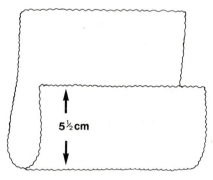

5½cm

31 Fold up one side of square
for purse

Purse

Knit a square 5½in × 5½in (14cm × 14cm). If using double knitting you will need about 36 stitches on the needles. Fold up one edge of the square 2¼in (5.5cm) (*fig 31*).

Using a contrasting colour and working in double crochet, join one side together starting at the fold; work up the side and continue up the side of the flap, along the top and down the other side (see *fig 32*). Make two button loops (see p 71) and sew on two small buttons.

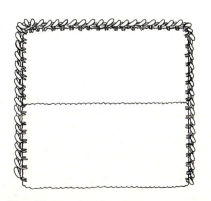

32 Double crochet in
contrasting colour around edge
of purse

Crochet bag on wooden handles

Make 32 Afghan squares in two colours. Crochet or stitch together into two pieces each four squares by four squares.

With right sides facing, stitch or crochet the two pieces together along the bottom and up both sides, leaving one and a half squares open from the top on both sides to form the gusset which allows the bag to open. Then attach the handles and lining as for the knitted bag on plywood handles (above).

Knitted bag on wooden handles

Knit 12 squares of various colours, $5\frac{1}{2}$in × $5\frac{1}{2}$in (14cm × 14cm), in double knitting.

Do this by casting on 36 stitches and knitting until you have a square.

Ladder stitch the squares to make an oblong piece of knitting, three squares by four squares. With right sides together, fold in half and stitch up $7\frac{1}{2}$in (19cm) of both sides (*fig 34*).

Slide one side of the top of the bag through the slit in one of the handles and hem stitch to the inside of the bag (*fig 35*). This will

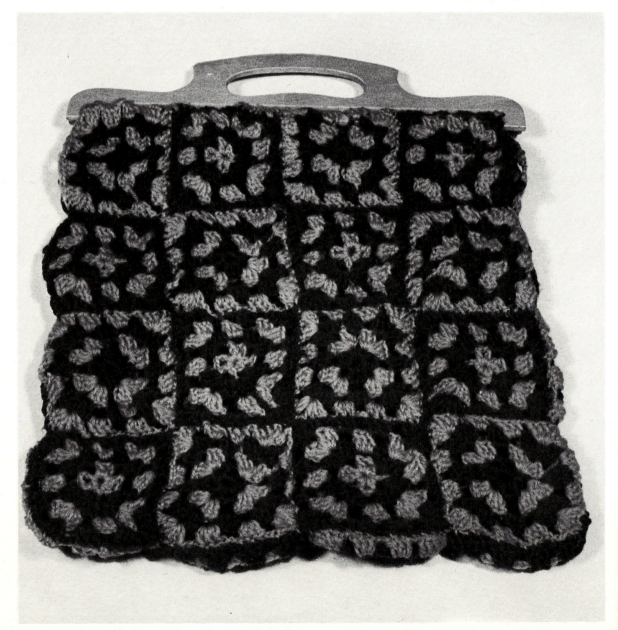

33 Crochet bag on wooden handles

automatically gather the top of the bag in. Repeat with other handle.

Cut a piece of lining material, preferably matching one of the colours used in the squares, to a size slightly larger than the bag.

Stitch up the sides the same distance as stitching on the bag.

Turn the bag the right side out and with raw edges of the lining turned inwards, slip the lining inside the bag. Ladder stitch the lining to the inside of the top of the bag and along each of the sides.

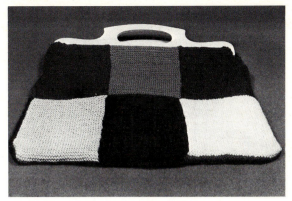

36 Knitted bag on wooden handles

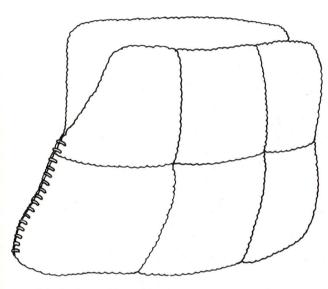

34 Stitched up sides of bag

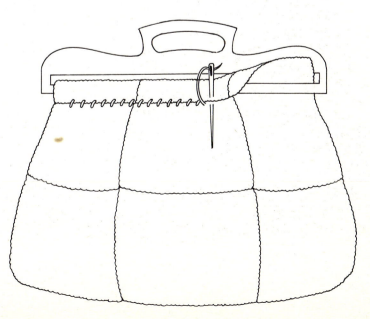

35 Attaching handle to bag on inside

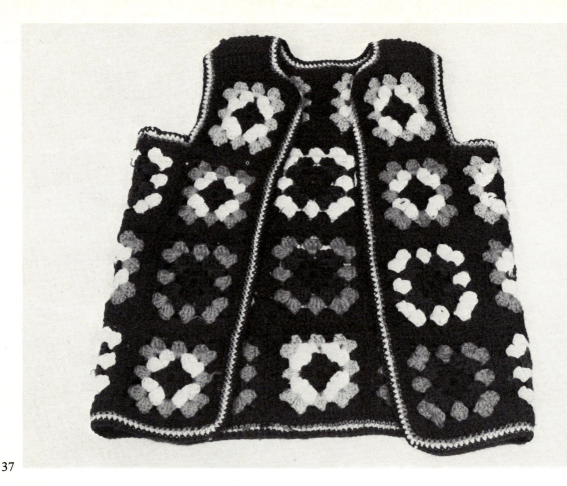

37

Child's waistcoat

Size Length 14½in (36cm)
    Chest 22in (56cm)

Make 25 Afghan squares, using the same colour for the fourth and last round on all the squares.

Stitch or crochet together seven squares for each of the two front pieces and eleven squares for the back (*fig 38*).

Left front
With right side facing, rejoin yarn to armhole side of the top square with a slip stitch.
3 ch, 10 tr, along the top of the square, which should bring you to the middle.
3 ch, turn, work another row of treble. Cast off.

Right front
With right side facing rejoin yarn to centre of top square.
3 ch, 10 tr, to end of square.
3 ch turn, work another row of treble. Cast off.

Back
With right side facing, join yarn on right edge of the top two squares.
3 ch, work 10 treble along top of first square.
3 ch, turn, work 2 more rows of treble. Cast off. Join yarn to centre of left-hand top square.
3 ch, 10 tr, along edge of square to the end.
3 ch, turn, work 2 more rows of treble.

This gives the shoulder shaping. With right sides together, stitch or crochet together the shoulder seam and the two side seams.

Rejoin the yarn at the centre bottom of the back with right side facing you. Work four rows of double crochet all the way round the outside edge. This can be done all in one colour or using a different colour for each row.

Work 4 rows of double crochet around each arm hole.

The waistcoat does not have any fastenings.

It should be fairly easy to modify this pattern to fit other sizes by adding more squares.

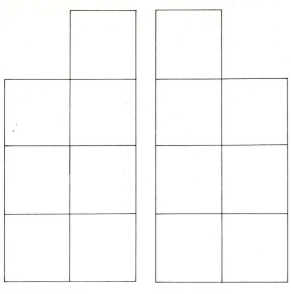

RIGHT FRONT   LEFT FRONT

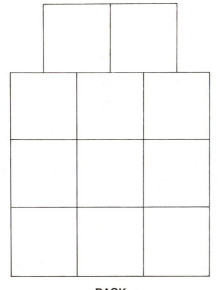

BACK

38 Arrangement of crochet
squares for waistcoat

Cushion cover

Decide upon the size of cushion and make enough squares for both sides. Stitch or crochet together the squares to make two pieces. Rejoin yarn to the edge of one and work rows of treble all the way round. Repeat on other side.

With right sides together, stitch or crochet the two pieces together on three sides.

As the Afghan square is fairly open work the cushion cover will need to be lined with material, picking out one of the colours used in the squares.

For instructions on how to make a cushion see p 18.

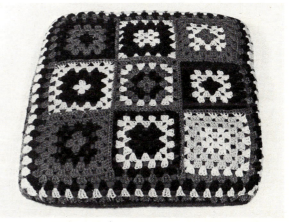

39 Cushion cover

FURTHER USEFUL INFORMATION: UNITED KINGDOM

The statutory provision of craft training facilities for the elderly and disabled is complemented by the services of a variety of voluntary and commercial organisations. While some provide training courses for instructors, others will advise individuals on suitable tools and materials. A further group can help craft workers with the sale of their work. All these services are outlined below. The suppliers listed all specialise to some extent in crafts supplies for the elderly or disabled.

The list of further reading is divided into sections relating to the different crafts described in the book, with a separate general section at the end.

HOW LOCAL AUTHORITIES CAN HELP

Under the Chronically Sick and Disabled Persons Act of 1970, county councils are empowered, but by no means obliged, to set up craft teaching facilities in day centres for the sick and the disabled.

The vague terms of this Act and the preceding National Assistance Act of 1948 have led to widely varying interpretations at the local level. Services are organised by the county councils, and information on craft teaching facilities in any particular area can be obtained from the county council's Social Services Department. Initial contact may be made through a social worker.

Most county councils support day centres or clubs for the disabled and elderly, with transport provisions and home visits for the housebound. Craft materials are often supplied by the county council's instructors, usually at reduced prices. Surrey County Council, for example, organises supplies at 10 per cent above cost. The same council will undertake the sale of craft work through its 'craft caravan' which visits local events. In Berkshire, on the other hand, sales are organised through the British Red Cross Society.

The disabled are allowed to earn £4 per week (£6 per week for single parents) before supplementary benefits are affected. Those receiving incapacity benefit can, if a doctor considers craft work to be therapeutically desirable, earn up to £10 per week before benefits fall. Without such medical approval, benefits are affected immediately. Further information about income benefits is given in the excellent *Disability Rights Handbook for 1978* published by the Disability Alliance and available from them at 65p including postage, at 5 Netherhall Gardens. London NW3.

Information about craft education evening and day classes for the disabled at adult education institutes can be obtained from the county council's education offices.

OTHER ORGANISATIONS AND WHAT THEY DO

British Association of Occupational Therapists
20 Rede Place, London W1. Tel 01-229 9738. *Most occupational therapists work within the National Health Service, and in recent years their systematic involvement in craft training has decreased. However, the occupational therapist may use craft teaching for medical purposes. The Association's monthly magazine often carries advertisements for craft materials. Occupational therapists remain closely involved with the training of voluntary workers for craft teaching work in day centres and clubs for the disabled and elderly.*

British Red Cross Society
6 Grosvenor Crescent, London SW1. Tel 01-235 7131. *The Hand Crafts Service of the Berkshire branch of the Red Cross operates the Helping Hand shop in Reading, selling craft work made by the area's disabled and elderly. Craftsmen receive payment for the goods before sale. Only high quality goods are accepted. A similar operation is run by the Oxford branch.*

Crafts Advisory Committee
12 Waterloo Place, London SW1. Tel 01-839 1917. *The CAC publishes several useful reference lists, including* Craft Societies in England and

Wales, Craft Shops and Galleries in England and Wales *and* Useful Addresses, a list of organisations and services likely to be of interest to craftsmen. *The bi-monthly magazine* Crafts *published by the CAC contains advertisements for crafts suppliers.*

Chest, Heart and Stroke Association
Tavistock House North, Tavistock Square, London WC1. Tel 01-387 3012. *'Stroke clubs' are organised for the disabled, where craft training is occasionally introduced.*

Disabled Living Foundation
346 Kensington High St, London W14. Tel 01-602 2491. *While concentrating its effort on the adaptation of living space to the needs of the disabled, the Foundation can advise on such matters as the adaptation of a sewing machine following disablement.*

Hand Crafts Advisory Association for the Disabled
103 Brighton Rd, Purley, Surrey. Tel 01-668 1411. *The Association's courses offer excellent instruction in craft teaching for groups of some dozen people. Courses are organised throughout the country, generally lasting one or two days, and are free to members. A twice-yearly bulletin, free to members, contains articles on crafts and information on equipment and new books. Membership costs £2.50 per annum at present. Many county councils belong.*

Homebound Craftsmen
25a Holland St, London W8. Tel 01-937 3924. *A charity organisation selling craft work by the elderly or disabled on a sale or return basis. Only work of the highest quality is accepted. A small sample of work should be sent to be examined for suitability. Articles are accepted from all over the country.*

Royal Association for Disability and Rehabilitation
25 Mortimer St, London W1. Tel 01-637 5400. *Formed by the amalgamation of the British Council for the Rehabilitation of the Disabled and the Central Council for the Disabled, the Association has a wide range of publications. A free list is available.*

Spastics Society
12 Park Crescent, London W1. Tel 01-636 5020. *The Recreation Department of the Society runs recreation courses throughout the country, with a craft element where suitable.*

SUPPLIERS OF CRAFT MATERIALS AND EQUIPMENT

Most of the materials mentioned in the book are available from ordinary high street shops: haberdasheries, department stores and DIY shops. The list of suppliers below is intended to help with those items not widely available, to give mail order firms for those who have difficulty in getting to a shopping centre, and also to provide details of companies who sell craft materials in bulk to local authorities, teachers of the disabled, etc.

There are two useful books which give addresses of craft suppliers. *Shopping by Post,* published by Exley Publications at £1.95, is obtainable from them at 63 Kingsfield Road, Watford, Herts (tel Watford 43892). It has a good section on hobbies and crafts, which includes suppliers of materials for embroidery, tapestry, knitting, crochet, soft toys, rug making and many other crafts. It also has an excellent section on aids for the disabled, with suppliers of numerous useful household items specially adapted for the disabled. *The Studio Vista Guide to Craft Suppliers* by Judy Allen, published by Cassell, is unfortunately out of print, but it is worth trying your local library for this as it has by far the most comprehensive list of suppliers.

Anything Left-Handed
65 Beak St, London W1. Tel 01-437 3910. *This shop sells some sixty items specially manufactured for the left-handed. They will supply a mail order catalogue on receipt of two 7p stamps. Articles for sale include left-handed corkscrews, knives and scissors. Stirex scissors, designed for those who cannot exert any pressure to cut, are now widely available from craft shops and haberdashers. Nottingham Handcraft Co (see below) supply them in bulk.*

Bullocks Sewing Machine Co

Lichfield Street, Wolverhampton. *This company will adapt their sewing machines for operation by mouth, to suit individual requirements.*

Carter and Parker Ltd

Gordon Mills, Guiseley, Leeds, West Yorkshire. Tel 0943 72264. *The company manufactures hand-knit yarns and large-print knitting and crochet patterns. Although unable to supply direct to individual members of the public, orders are accepted from county councils, welfare services and teachers of the disabled.*

Dryad Handicrafts and Needlecrafts

PO Box 38, Northgates, Leicester. Tel 0533 50405. *General crafts suppliers, dealing with both educational establishments and members of the public. Two free mail order catalogues are available, including information on their stool frames for caning.*

Dunlicraft Ltd

Magna Rd, South Wigston, Leicester. Tel 0533 786331. *A very wide range of crafts materials, supplied to hospitals, social services and the retail trade. Teachers wishing to order goods should obtain a covering letter of authorisation from the employing authority.*

Dycem Ltd

Parkway Trading Estate, 15 Minto Rd, Bristol. Tel 0272 559921. *Manufacturers of non-slip materials, including plastic-coated trays which can be tilted without the contents falling off. Small orders from members of the public are not accepted.*

Goodlad and Goodlad

Esplanade, Lerwick, Shetland. 0595 3797. *This company will supply a Shetland knitting pad by post.*

Homecraft Supplies Ltd

27 Trinity Rd, London SW17. 01-672 1789. *An illustrated catalogue details Homecraft's wide range of craft materials, sold both wholesale to bulk buyers and retail to individual members of the public. They have a mail order service.*

The Needlewoman Shop

146–148 Regent Street, London W1. Tel 01-734 1727. *This shop has a good stock of materials and equipment for sewing, embroidery, tapestry, rug making, knitting and crochet. They have a mail order service with a catalogue.*

Nottingham Handcraft Company

Melton Rd, West Bridgford, Nottingham. Tel 0602 234251. *Crafts suppliers dealing only with bulk orders to social service departments, educational establishments, hospitals and other organisations.*

Singer Co (UK) Ltd

Consumer Products Division, 255 High Street, Guildford. Tel 0483 71144. *This division of Singer will adapt their electric sewing machines for operation by knee, elbow, or chin.*

Smit and Co Ltd

99 Walnut Tree Close, Guildford, Surrey. Tel 0483 33113. *Cane importers and crafts suppliers whose main trade is wholesale supply of articles for handicraft work to organisations.*

Weavers' Shop

Royal Wilton Carpet Factory, King St, Wilton, Wiltshire. Tel 072274 2441. *A shop providing personal service and a mail order service to members of the public, supplying yarn in hanks and carpet thrums. A price list and samples will be sent on receipt of 15p in stamps.*

FURTHER READING

Canvas embroidery

T. H. de Dillmont, *Encyclopedia of Needlework*, Philadelhia, Pa., Running Press, 1955

Anne Dyer and Valerie Duthoit, *Canvas Work from the Start*, London, Bell, 1972

Nancy Hobbs, *Imaginative Canvas Embroidery*, London, Pitman, 1976

Mary Thomas, *Dictionary of Embroidery Stitches*, London, Hodder, 1934

Anna Wilson, *Enjoying Embroidery*, London, Batsford, 1975

Soft toys

Gladys and Kathryn Greenaway, *Soft Toy Making*, London, Pelham, 1973

Anna Griffiths, *Felt Gifts and Toys*, London, Batsford, 1974

Margaret Hutchings, *Making and Using Finger Puppets*, London, Mills and Boon, 1973

Margaret Hutchings, *Modern Soft Toy Making*, London, Mills and Boon, 1959 (*out of print, but worth getting from your local library*)

G. P. Jones, *Easy-to-make Dolls with Nineteenth-Century Costumes*, New York, Dover Publications, 1977

Vivian Rees, *Making Nursery Rhyme Soft Toys*, London, Studio Vista, 1975

R. L. Sarigny, *Good Design in Soft Toys*, London, Mills and Boon, 1971

Knitting and crochet

Pam Dawson, ed, *A Complete Guide to Crochet*, London, Marshall Cavendish, 1976

Nicki Hitz Edson and Arlene Stimmel, *Creative Crochet*, London, Pitman, 1974

Knitting Dictionary, London, Conde Nast, 1971

Eve de Negri, *Knitting and Crochet in Easy Steps*, London, Studio Vista, 1977

Chair caning

Margery Brown, *Cane and Rush Seating*, London, Batsford, 1976

Barbara Maynard, *Cane Seating* (leaflet), Enfield, Dryad Press, nd

Other useful books

Coping with Disablement, London, Consumers' Association, 1974; revised edn 1976 (section on pastimes, pp 190–5)

Disabled Living Foundation, Information Service for the Disabled issues a series of lists of aids and equipment, societies, etc. List 6 *Leisure Activities* (and Appendix 1) gives relevant information on hobbies and pastimes, clubs, music, sport and holidays, among other things

Ruth Elliot, *Life and Leisure for the Physically Handicapped*, London, Elek, 1971 (Chapter 6, Leisure and holidays, pp 105–14)

Sydney Foott, *Handicapped at Home*, London, Design Centre in association with the Disabled Living Foundation, 1977 (Chapter 9, Recreation, pp 52–9)

Brenda Morton, *Hobbies for the Housebound*, London, Mills and Boon, 1961

Philip Nichols, *Living with a Handicap*, London, Priory Press, 1973 (Chapter 12, Leisure, pp 114–25)

E. E. Rogers and B. M. Stevens, *Dressmaking for the Disabled*, Association of Occupational Therapists, 1966

Oxford Regional Health Authority, *Equipment for the Disabled* (a series of booklets). No 6 in the series, Leisure and gardening, contains extensive lists of addresses of various leisure societies, details of equipment available and addresses of manufacturers. Leisure interests covered include music and art, sewing, cards and other games, sports and gardening. Orders for this and other titles in the series should be sent to Equipment for the Disabled, 2 Foredown Drive, Portslade, Sussex.

Practical Aids for the Disabled, London British Red Cross Society, nd

FURTHER USEFUL INFORMATION: UNITED STATES

Government provision for the disabled and the aged in the USA is implemented by the Social and Rehabilitation Service of the US Department of Health, Education and Welfare (3rd and Independence Streets SW, Washington, DC 20201, tel: (202) 963-3155). The Bureau of Education for the Handicapped, at the US Office of Education (7th and Dependence Streets SW, Washington, DC 20202, tel: (202) 963-5925) gives support to states for training teachers of the handicapped, for research and demonstration projects and also for the provision of instructional materials and the production and distribution of media and materials for the handicapped. It also gives aid to states for schools services for the handicapped.

OTHER ORGANISATIONS AND WHAT THEY DO

The Arthritis Foundation

1212 Avenue of the Americas, New York, NY 10036. Tel (212) 757-7600. *Through its local chapters throughout the country, the Foundation provides community services to patients and their families as well as seeking to improve treatment techniques and encouraging research. They publish handbooks for patients and informative pamphlets and brochures on arthritis, and a list of publications is available on request.*

Boy Scouts of America – Scouting for the Handicapped Division and Girl Scouts of the USA – Scouting for the Handicapped Girl Program

N. Brunswick, NJ 08902. Tel (201) 249-6000 (Boy Scouts) and 830 Third Avenue, New York, NY 10022. Tel: (212) 751-6900 (Girl Scouts). *These two organisations encourage the inclusion of handicapped young people in their regular activities but have also established special packs, troops and posts at institutions and homes for the handicapped. They place emphasis on job preparation for the disabled, and their many recreational activities include crafts.*

Federation of the Handicapped Inc

211 West 14th Street, New York, NY 10011. Tel: (212) 242-9050. *This is a private, non-profit organisation whose purpose is the vocational rehabilitation of the disabled. Their programs include PATH (Personal Aides for the Homebound), High School Homebound and Training Services.*

Goodwill Industries of America

9200 Wisconsin Avenue, Washington, DC 20014. Tel (301) 530-6500. *Founded in 1902, this widespread organisation provides vocational rehabilitation and training for employment.*

International Association of Rehabilitation Facilities, Inc

5530 Wisconsin Avenue 955, Washington, DC 20015. Tel (301) 654-5882. *The Association has 700 medically orientated rehabilitation centers and sheltered workshops. They hold educational seminars throughout the year and publish a bimonthly newsletter.*

Muscular Dystrophy Associations of America Inc

1790 Broadway, New York, NY 10019. Tel (212) 586-0808. *A voluntary health organisation with over 300 chapters throughout the US. Programs include patient services, recreational*

programs and community clinics in large cities.

National Association of the Physically Handicapped Inc

6473 Grandville Avenue, Detroit, Michigan 48228. Tel (313) 271-0160. *Over 1000 members of the Association belong to autonomous local chapters, whose programs include recreation and sports activities.*

National Congress of Organisations of the Physically Handicapped Inc

7611 Oakland Avenue, Minneapolis, Minn. 55423. Tel (612) 861-2162. *Representing the physically handicapped and their organisations, the Congress serves as an advisory, co-ordinating and representative body in promoting employment opportunities, legislation and equal rights, social activities and rehabilitation. They publish a roster of clubs of the physically handicapped.*

National Easter Seal Society for Crippled Children and Adults

2023 West Ogden Avenue, Chicago, Illinois 60612. Tel (312) 243-8400. *Aims to help the disabled and their families to find and make effective use of resources to develop their abilities. The Society also assists in the development of community resources for the disabled, and their programs include sheltered workshops, homebound employment and pre-school programs.*

National Industries for the Blind

1455 Broad Street, Bloomfield, New Jersey 07003. Tel (201) 338-3804. *A non-profit corporation whose aim is to promote gainful employment for the blind, they run 83 workshops for the blind in 35 different states. Their Rehabilitation Services Division runs training programmes.*

Sister Kenny Institute

1800 Chicago Avenue, Minneapolis, Minn. 55404. Tel (612) 333-4251. *A non-profit hospital and rehabilitation center founded in 1942 and specialising in the rehabilitation of the disabled. Programs include courses and workshops in community hospitals and nursing homes.*

SUPPLIERS OF CRAFT MATERIALS AND EQUIPMENT

Many of the materials mentioned in this book may be bought locally in craft shops, needlework shops and variety stores, but for those who have difficulty in reaching retail outlets or in finding supplies locally, the following mail-order catalogues are recommended:

Margaret A. Boyd *The Mail-Order Crafts Catalogue* Radnor, Pa., Chilton Book Company, 1973. $12.50

Deborah Lippman & Paul Collin *Craft Sources: The Ultimate Catalogue For Craftspeople* New York, M. Evans & Co. Inc., 1975, $12.50; $5.95 paper.

Joseph Rosenbloom (ed) *Craft Supplies Supermarket* (Finder's Guide Series No. 2) Willits, Calif., Oliver Press, 1974. $3.95.

Catalogues of needlework supplies are also obtainable from: Merribee Needlecraft Company at 1297 Massachusetts Avenue, Arlington, Massachusetts 02174 and from Lee Ward at 1200 St. Charles Street, Elgin, Illinois 60120.

Self-Help Aids and General Supplies

Tables and other furniture

Work tables, constructed without the usual apron front and with a height clearance of 30½ inches, to enable a wheelchair to be placed in close proximity, can be obtained from: J. A. Preston Corporation, 71 Fifth Avenue, New York, NY 10003. Call toll-free (800) 221-2425. In New York call collect (212) 255-8484. In Canada: J. A. Preston of Canada Ltd., 3220 Wharton Way, Mississauga, Ontario L4X 2C1. Call toll-free 1-800-261-2032. In Toronto area call 416-625-5959. Catalogue available on request.

Left-handed scissors

A wide selection of left-handed pinking shears, embroidery scissors, sewing scissors and dressmaker's bent trimmers, of use to craftspeople without the use of their right hand can be obtained mail-order from: The Left Hand Inc., 140 West 22nd Street, New York, NY 10011. Catalogue available on request. Telephone orders are accepted for credit card orders with American Express ($15.00 minimum), Master Charge ($10.00 minimum) and Bank Americard/VISA ($5.00 minimum) on (212) 675-6265 but no collect calls.

Needle threaders

Automatic needle threaders are available from: Reston Manufacturing Company, Naugatuck, Connecticut 06770.

Wire needle threaders combined with magnifying glasses are supplied by Scovill-Dritz Manufacturing Company, Spartanburg, South Carolina 20301.

Yarn threaders are available from Muriel's Needlecraft Company Inc., P.O. Box 12, Fitchburg, Massachusetts 01420.

Easy-to-work plastic mesh

This fabric which is easy to hold and drop a needle into is available from: Columbia-Minerva Corporation, 295 Fifth Avenue, New York, NY 10016.

Ready counted-thread fabrics

These fabrics which take the hard work out of pattern designing are supplied by:

Art Needlework Treasure Trove, P.O. Box 2440, Grand Central Station, New York, NY 10017.

Ball Of Yarn, 1208 Gordon Street, Charlotte, North Carolina 28205.

Needlecraft Shop, 4501 Van Nuys Boulevard, Sherman Oaks, California 91403.

Selma's Art Needlework, 1645 Second Avenue, New York, NY 10028.

FURTHER READING

Cora Bodkin et al *Crafts For Your Leisure Years*, Boston, Mass., Houghton Mifflin, 1976. $14.95; $7.95 paper

Jane G. Kay *Crafts For The Very Disabled And Handicapped: For All Ages* Springfield, Ill., Charles C. Thomas, 1977. $15.50

Elaine Gould & Loren Gould *Crafts For The Elderly* Springfield, Ill., Charles C. Thomas, 1976. $9.75

Regina Hurlburt *Left-Handed Needlepoint* New York, Van Nostrand Reinhold Company, 1972. $4.50 paper

Carole Robbins Myers *A Primer Of Left-*

Handed Embroidery New York, Charles Scribners' Sons, 1974. $8.95

Iris Rosenthal *Not So Nimble Needlework Book* New York, Grosset & Dunlap, Inc., 1977

Elaine Slater *The New York Times Book Of Needlepoint For Left-Handers* New York, Quadrangle/The New York Times Book Co. Inc., 1973, $14.95

The craft books listed here have been specially selected for the advice they offer to the craftsperson with manual dexterity problems. If you have difficulty in reaching a book store to buy these or the many other general craft books which deal with your craft interest, write to: The Unicorn, Box 645R, Rockville, Md 20851. This firm produces a very extensive catalog of books for craftspersons and attempts to carry all craft books in print in the United States, as well as importing some craft books from abroad.

The following books are recommended for housebound people who may wish to supplement their income by making craft work for sale. Needless to say, you should have reached a very proficient stage in your chosen craft, before attempting to market it:

Patricia Brent *Craft Careers* New York, Franklin Watts Inc., 1977. $4.47

Crafts As Business: A Bibliography New York, The American Crafts Council, 1975. $3.95

Crafts Business Bookshelf: An Annotated Bibliography For Craftsmen And Retailers New York, The American Crafts Council, 1977. $4.90

Handicrafts And Home Business, SBB No. 1 and *Selling By Mail Order* SBB No. 3, both obtainable on request from: The Small Business Administration (SBA), Washington, DC 20416

Michael Scott *Craft Business Encyclopedia* New York, Harcourt Brace Jovanovitch Inc., 1977. $10.00

George Wettlaufer & Nancy Wettlaufer *Craftsman's Survival Manual: Making A Full Or Part-Time Living From Your Crafts* Englewood Cliffs, NJ, Prentice-Hall Inc., 1974. $9.95; $3.45 paper

Leta W. Clark *How To Make Money With Your Crafts* New York, William Morrow. $6.95